Foodie wanna be

Contents

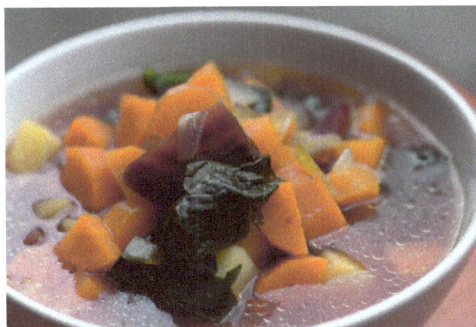

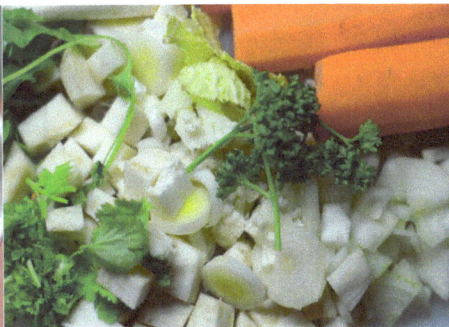

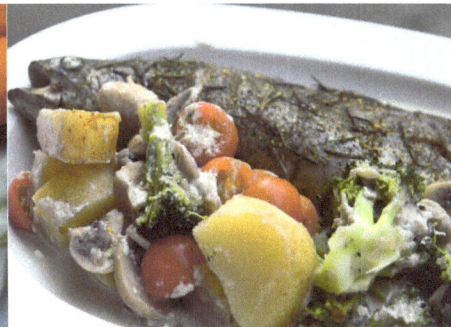

Acknowledgements

To be honest this is one of the hardest... to write acknowledgement. First of all, I have never done it and second of all it also takes longer than any of the pages within the book. Thinking why, well I shall say since you try to be grateful to those who are the closest to you no matter if friends; family or whoever is important to you and who has supported you at least somehow. Sometimes the tears in your eyes are another thing which slows you down.

So to my remarkable wife, we have been married just of one year after 2 outstanding years long relationship but you still continue to amaze me. It has never been really easy how we met how we cope and what we can expect from our life given to our completely different cultures but nevertheless I think I can say I'm blessed to spend portion of my life with you, to have you as a mother to my kid(s?), my partner, chinese translator :-) and best friend.

To my son, Samuel, I can't wait to see what amazing things has life in store for you and I just want you to know that watching you grow is without doubt going to be one of my life's greatest joy. Surely you may expect obstacles in your life but this is you know just the way it is done. We will make sure to do our best to eliminate such. A matter of remark just to let you know we've been working on this book with your mum when you were still safely wrapped inside your mummy's belly. To be really precise at time of writting you were three weeks yet to be delivered (datestamp 16.03.2014)

To my parents, who do not speak english and unlikely I'm going to translate this to them, though they will certainly have one copy of this book since I don't really know how to express my feelings face to face and I don't like to melt!. I couldn't wish more from life concerning parents. I can seriously just pray I'm going to be the same caring and loving as you were to me. Actually to equel them I should do better than them since my position is much easier than they were 30 years ago.

To whoever who bought a copy of this book. We shall express our thank you and we hope that you will find it usefull on the way to fullfill your dreams whatever they are.

Getting started

Thank you for buying our publication we believe it will enrich your current gastronomy collection.

You see, food is everything. We live a life of being someone who thinks about food every single time. We actually live to eat, not eat to live! Shall you be on the same page? Very well then!

We aim to choose receipes which are healthy, fast and easy to prepare. Right in this order. What we consider healthy nowadays is very different from what earlier generation believed to be healthy. There was a time for example where meatless dish was considered to be deficient in essential nutrients and high-fat fried food was on daily menu. Nowadays we know that there is nothing wrong with vegetarian diet and that too many fried food can raise our cholesterol levels and increase our risk of having a heart attack. We've never been so well informed in fact there are so much information out there that it is very easy to become completely overhelmed and unable to distinguish between ideas that turns out to be fancy at times and those solid practical ideas. We think it is good to mention that this publication was not prepared with cooperation with nutrition specialist so all ideas and thoughts in this book are ours and as such subjective, you shouldn't simply follow them especially if you are allergic to some specific food or suffering some medical problem.

But still while listing through what we've written down we hope that our fusion between asian and european cuisine creates tasty dishes rich in nutrition and at the same time having an eye appeal as well. They are full of vegetable and light meat such as poultry or seafood. So don't be afraid as this is not a diet type of book you will have to strictly follow. This is just to show you other healtier alternatives to those dishes you may be well used to cook already. As previously stated we focus not only to have these dishes healthy but fast and easy to prepare as well which goes hand to hand with recent modern lifestyle. If we say fast we've set a deadline of maxium 30 minutes spent on preparation.

Every healthy diet should have a good supply of following basic food groups:

- Carbohydrates
let's distinguish between those simple which can be broken down quickly in the body such as those found in cakes, candies and other sugary food and those complex which are therefore longer-lasting energy source such as whole wheat bread, brown rice, etc. Guess which type you should eat more.

- Fats
not all fats are bad! Unsaturated fats found in fish, soybean oil, peanut oil and olive oil are indeed good for us. Bad guy to limit here is saturated fat - the one which tend to clog your arteries that can be found in meat such as pork or dairy. So try to limit this as much as you can.

- Protein
is essential for body development and can be found in meat, poultry, fish, dairy product, eggs and beans or nuts.

However there other things you should include if you are really up to live life healtier. You should consider drinking more water, which helps to carry nutrients around the body, digestion, cleans and hydrates the body. Limit alcohol intake (especially tough task down here in Czech republic !!!). Restict your intake of caffeine. Do you need special ingredients to eat healthy? Do you need any special equipment to prepare and cook healthy dishes? Not at all. The recipes in this book use the most common ingredients you can find and the usual basic kitchenware will do.

We are hoping in reminding you that eating at home should be more common than eating out. It's fun and it takes just up to 30 minutes to prepare a dish which is tastier, healtier and could be more economical as well than eating out. We wish that you will enjoy cooking for yourself since it is an incredible experience, which is slowly to be forgotten in shade of empty international food chains.

Relax and have fun !

Main's / Light bites

These recipes are light in every sense. Not only they are served in a relatively small, easy to digest portions, but they are also low in fat. In visual terms they are, mostly, immensely satisfying thanks to the perfect presentation of my wife's asian cooking passion.

Chinese cabbage in oyster sauce with glass noodles

Chinese cabbage with oyster sauce has a sweet flavor and is loaded with vitamins and minerals, the oyster sauce just enhanced the light taste of Chinese cabbage.

Cabbage, one of the oldest vegetables, continues to be a dietary staple and an inexpensive food. It is easy to grow, tolerates the cold, and keeps well. And, it tastes good. Cabbage provides multiple health benefits. Cabbage is rich in Vitamin C (an antioxidant) and fiber. People who frequently eat cabbage and other cruciferous vegetables may help reduce their risk of certain cancers such as colon and rectal cancer. Serving size of 84 g of cabbage has 15 calories, 0 g of fat, 10 mg of sodium, 2 g of carbohydrate, 1 g of dietary fiber, 1 g of sugars and 1 g of protein.

Ingredients:

- ginger (you will need only few slices)
- garlic (3-4 cloves) - chopped
- chinese cabbage (medium size)
- oyster sauce (5 table spoon)

Method:

Heat pot with a bit of oil, one table spoon will do. You may use olive oil or ordinary sunflower oil. Put ginger slices and chopped garlic into pot and fry till golden brown. Add chinese cabbage and stir gently, add oyster sauce and salt to taste. Once chinese cabbage is cooked (check whether it is soft already) add your last ingredient which is glass noodles. Turn off the gas and return in few minutes. Your dish will be ready.

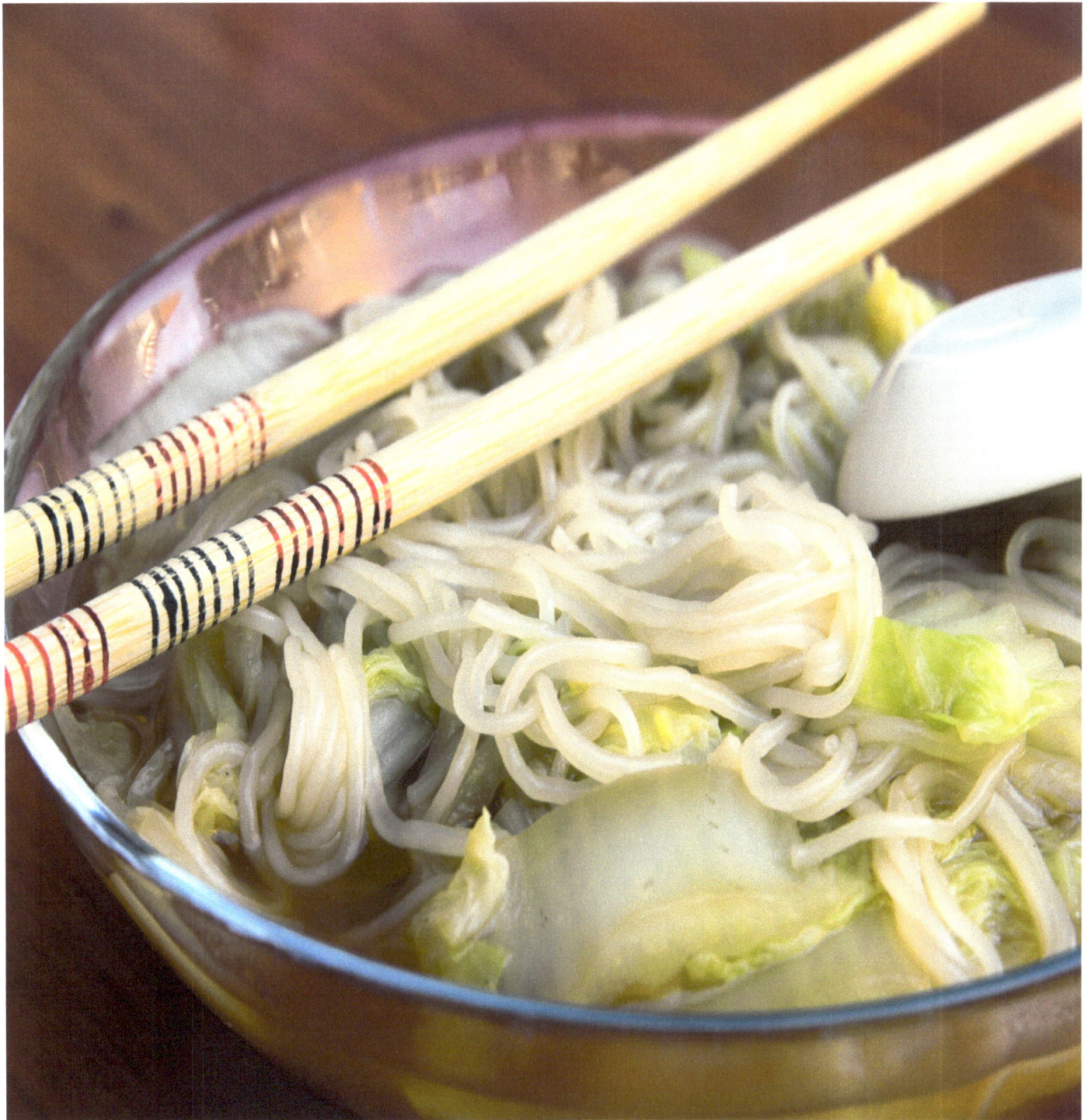

Wonton noodles with egg

Wonton noodles is a type of thin egg noodles easily accessible in any asian grocery shop. To accompany them we use eggs. Eggs are a great source of high quality protein with few calories. One whole egg has 5.5 grams of protein with only 68 calories. Eggs contain choline, which is important, especially since our bodies cannot produce enough of it.

Ingredients:

- egg noodles
- 1 teaspoon of sesame oil
- 2 tablespoons of soy sauce
- 1 teaspoon of dark soy sauce
- 2 etaspoons of oyster sauce
- eggs

Method:

Boil egg noodles till soft, at the same time fry eggs. Mix oil with all the other sauces onto the plate. Once egg noodles are soft enough drain the water and mix the noodles with the mixed sauces. Serve with fried egg nicely topping the plate. If you want, you can garnish the plate using spring onion or fresh parsley.

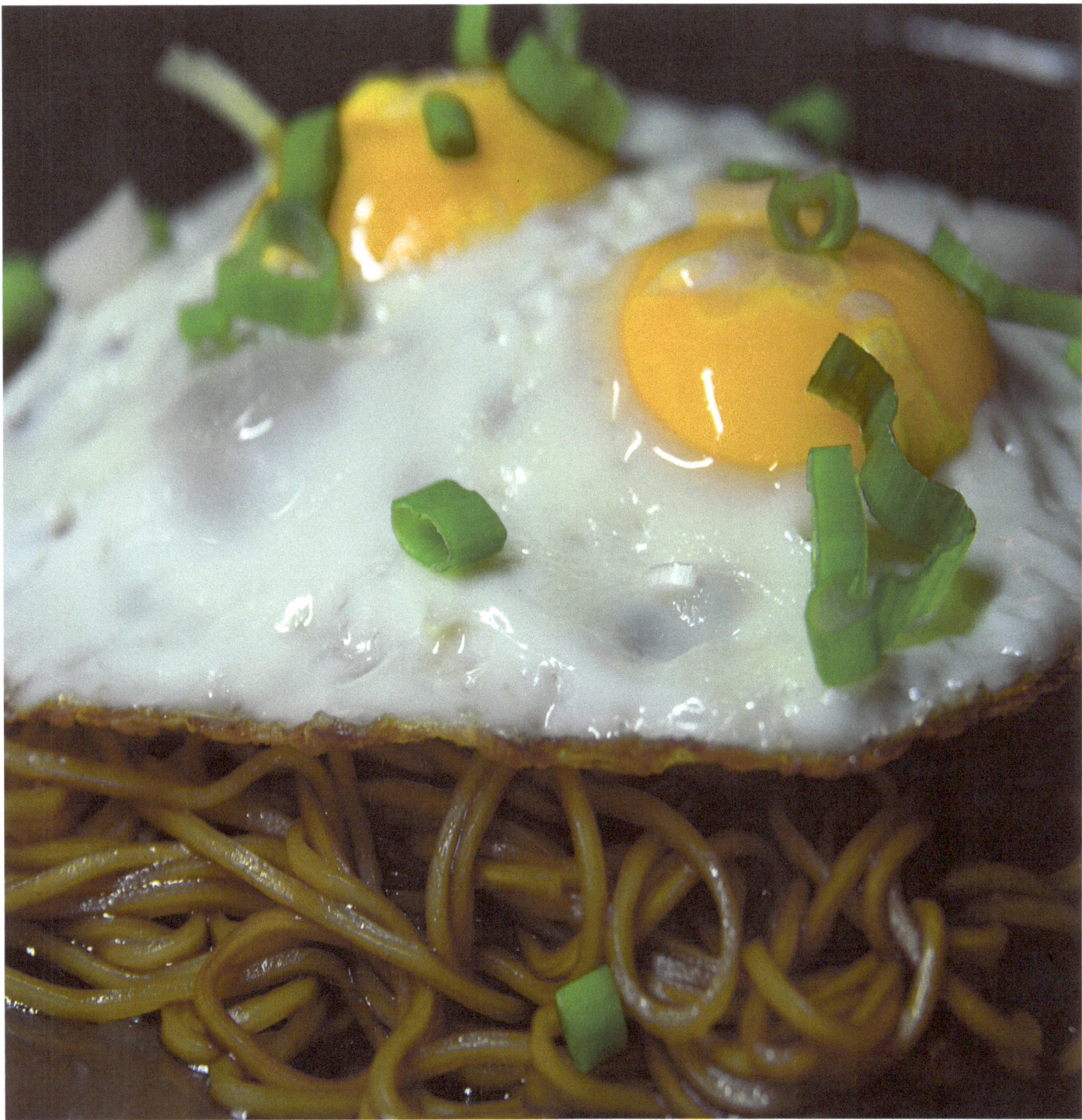

Curry white amur fish

White amur is an unusual fish which as an adult feeds almost exclusively on aquatic macrophytes. Its meat is white and tender and though this fish is not predator it is not fatty as usual freshwater fishes of similar kind such as carp.

Ingredients:

- 1 packet of curry fish paste
- white amur fish (freshwater fish of any kind will do)
- 1 big onion, chopped into pieces
- 1 tomato (if available)

Method:

Heat pan with 1 tablespoon of oil. Add in chopped big onion and stir fry till it turn slightly 'golden brown'. Add in curry fish paste and continue to stir the mixture of onion & paste for a minute. Add in a fish. Add a cup of water and let it simmer until the fish is done. Add in tomatoes followed by salt and a pinch of sugar to taste. Ensure that the fish is cooked well and serve with rice.

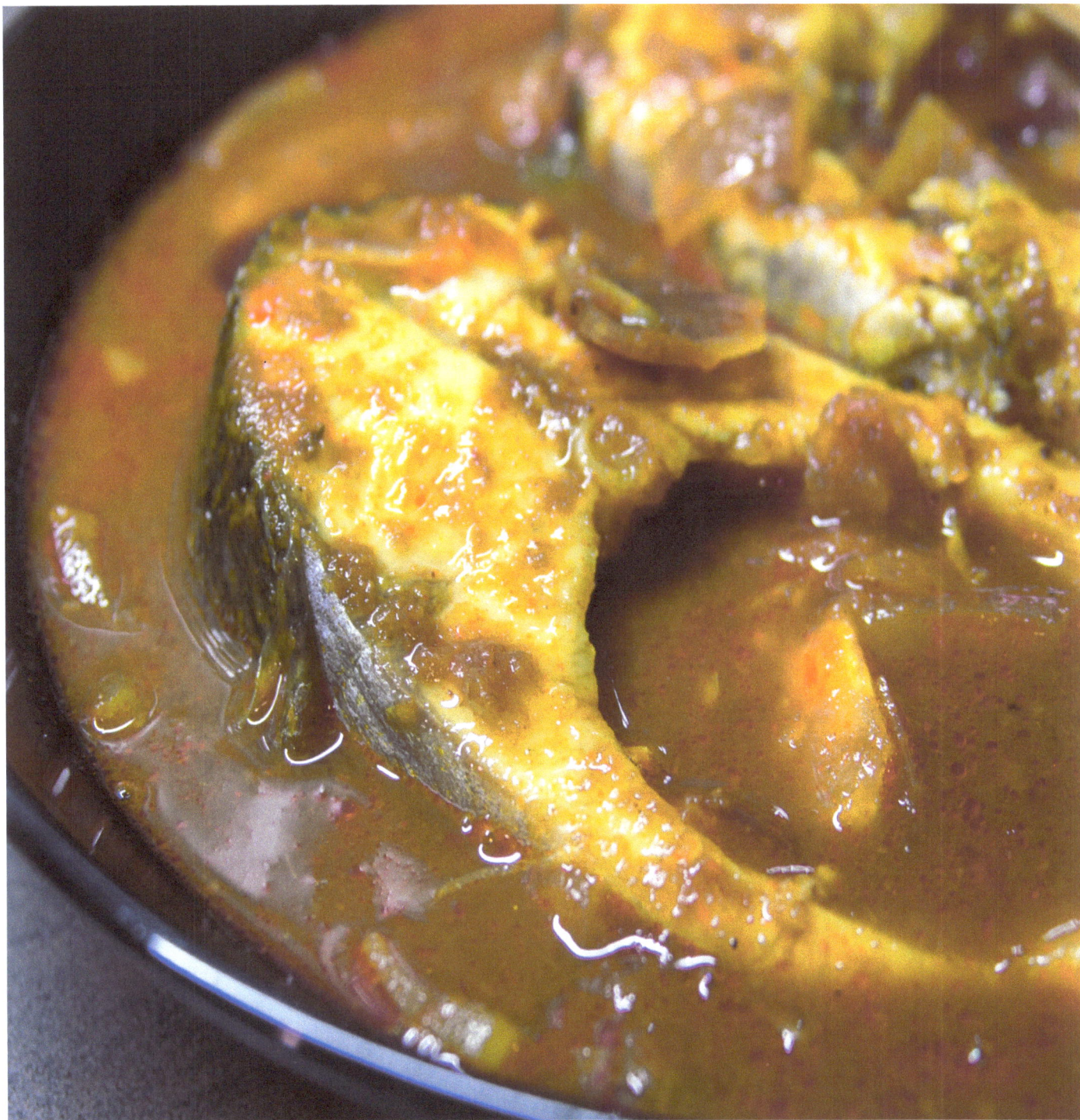

Salmon tartare

Light, fresh and easy, salmon tartare is sure to be a hit with fish fans. Use only the best fresh salmon fillets to make the tartare - the fish really is the star of the show here.

Ingredients:

- 1 large onion
- dill
- olive oil
- 1 lemon
- white pepper
- tablespoon of caper
- 300 g of fresh salmon fillet

Method:

Cut the salmon to as tiny pieces as you can and put into non-metal bowl. Chop the following ingredients into small pieces and put them all into the bowl with salmon: Onion, dill, caper. Squeeze lemon juice all over it and put a pinch or two of white pepper. Now stir with your hand the whole mixture untill all is nicely blended. Once mixture is prepared put it aside but not to the fridge as the taste will be richer when left outside. Toast the bread and serve while bread is still warm. Desirable taste is when you still can taste the fish so don't put much of any other ingredients as we indeed don't want to kill the fish taste.

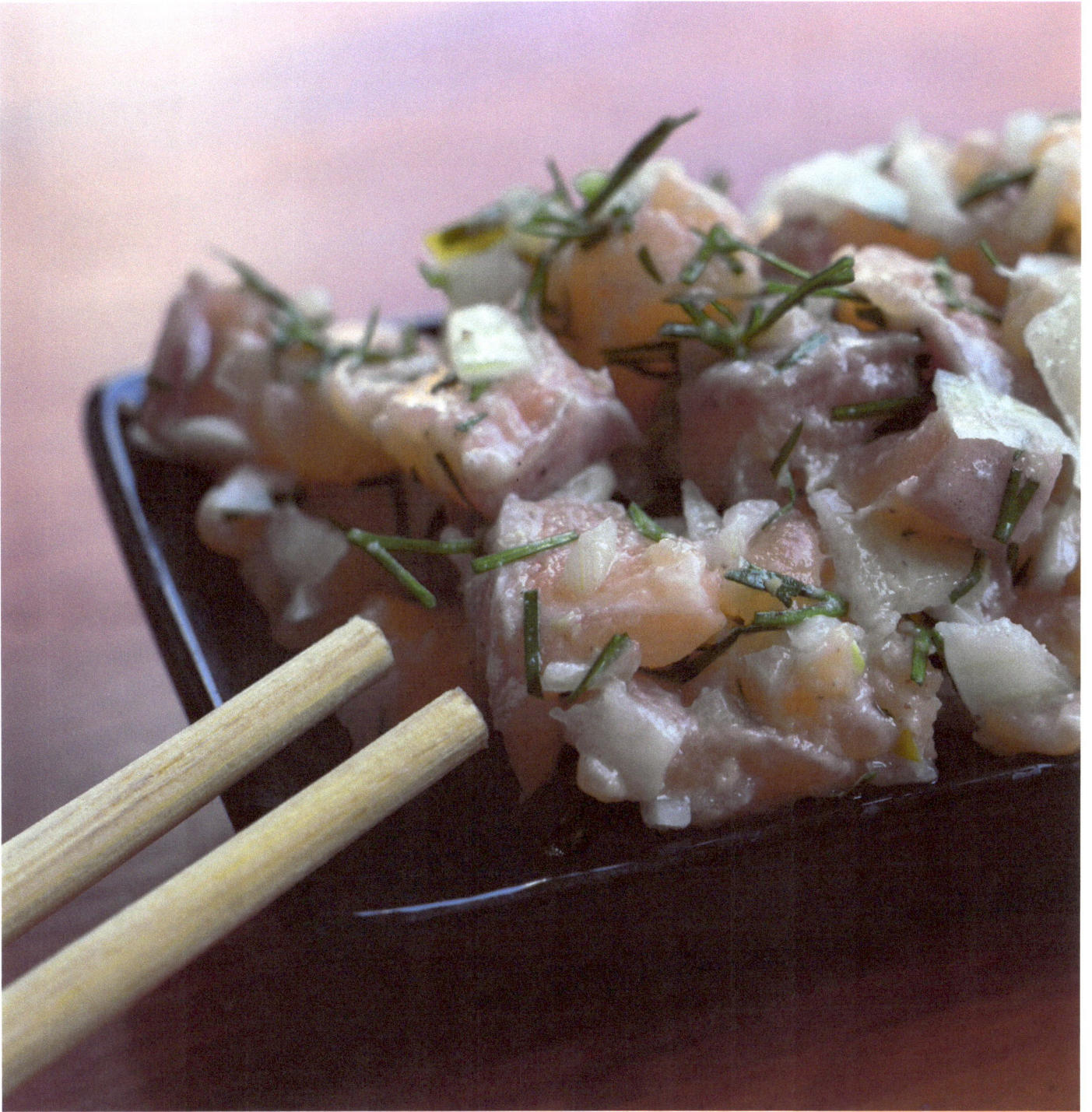

Brocoli with garlic sauce

You can without worries make this for the "big kid" in your life - husband. No matter how he hates veggies, but if he coo-coo for Asian flavors that perk up this crisp tender, nutritional packed veg!

Ingredients:

- 1 large bunch of fresh broccoli
- 3 large garlic cloves, chopped
- 1/2 cup fat-free, low-sodium beef or vegetable broth
- 1 tablespoon low-sodium soy sauce
- 1 tablespoon cornstarch
- 1 tablespoon brown sugar or sugar substitute
- 1 teaspoon sesame oil
- 1 tablespoon canola or corn oil
- 3-4 scallions, thinly sliced

Method:

Trim broccoli and cut into florets. Peel stalk with a vegetable peeler and slice thinly. Set aside. In a medium bowl, stir garlic, broth, soy sauce, cornstarch, sugar or sugar substitute, and sesame oil. Heat a large skillet over high heat and add the canola or corn oil. When the oil is hot, carefully add the broccoli. Cook 3-4 minutes, stirring continuously until the broccoli begins to brown slightly. Reduce the heat to medium and add 1/4 cup of water. Cover and cook 3-4 additional minutes until the broccoli begins to soften. Pour sauce over broccoli, cook 2-3 minutes longer until the broccoli is tender-crisp and the sauce thickens. Sprinkle with scallions and serve immediately.

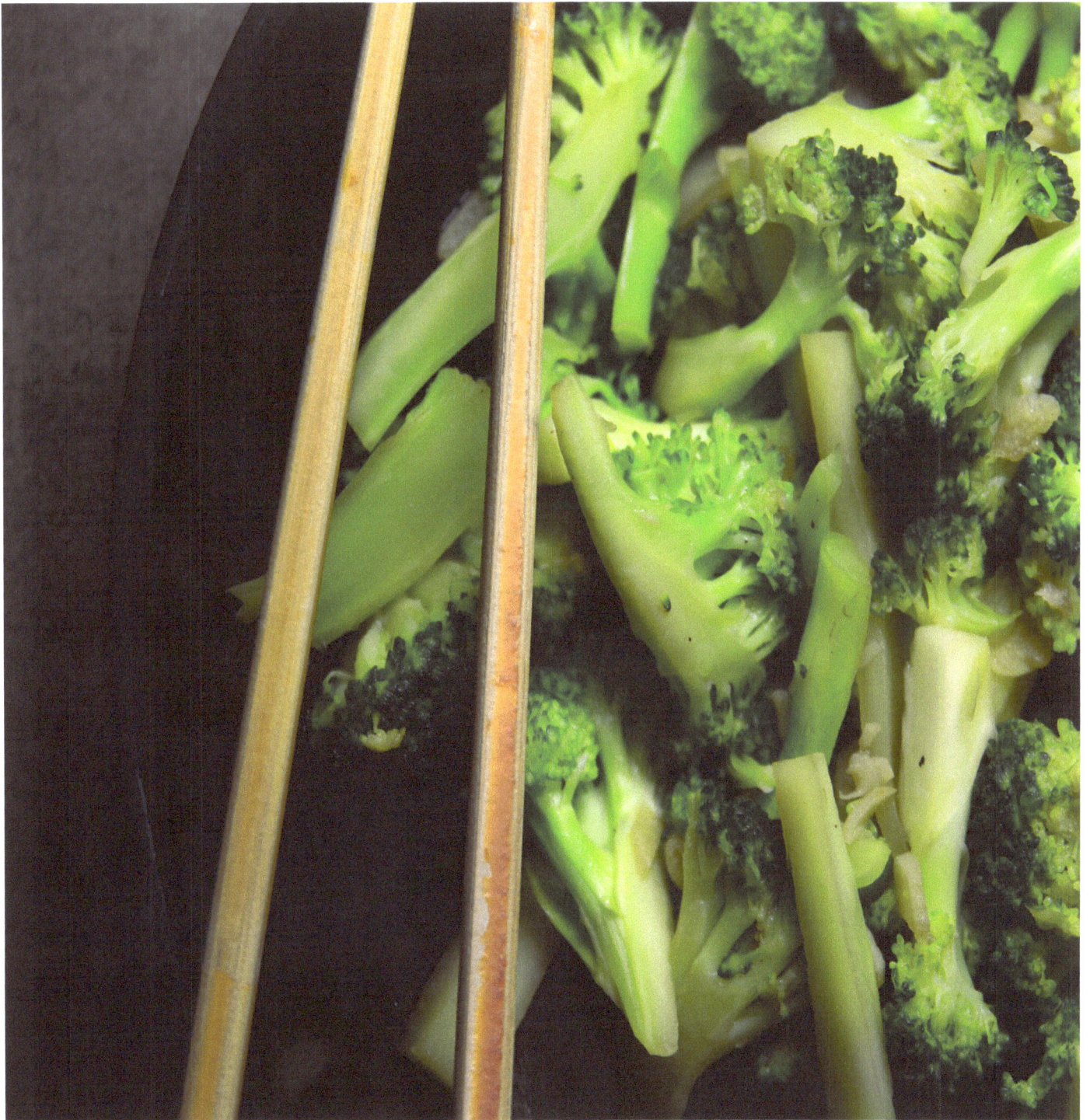

Basic sushi - salmon and avocado

Fresh, tasty and nutritious, salmon and avocado sushi is easy to make at home. Should this be your fish sushi recipe don't be affraid you can do that. Thankfully sushi is not a particularly fattening food. While the rice in sushi contains a fair amount of carbohydrates, sushi can be eaten without rice (as sashimi) and in moderation, even a standard sushi item can be a healthy treat without breaking the calorie bank. However keep in mind that the more rice you eat less this can be considered low caloric food.

Ingredients:

- 2 cups Japanese sushi rice
- 6 tablespoons rice wine vinegar
- 6 pieces of dry seaweed
- 2 avocado
- 150 g of smoked salmon, cut into long strips
- wasabi paste
- soy sauce

Method:

Should you be lucky enough you will have rice cooker. So you just put rice in with water and let it cook. Since rice must be slightly dry as vinegar will be added later don't put much of water just a bit more than rice itself. Immediately after rice is cooked, mix in rice vinegar to the hot rice. Then let it cool. Place a sheet of seaweed on bamboo mat and put a thin layer of cool rice on the seaweed. Leave at least a centimeter top and bottom edge of the seaweed uncovered. This is for easier sealing later. Arrange avocado and smoked salmon to the rice. Position them about 2 cm away from the bottom edge of the seaweed.Slightly wet the top edge of the seaweed. Roll from bottom to the top edge with the help of the bamboo mat tightly. Combine the soy sauce and wasabi in a small serving bowl. Cut roll into equal pieces (if really cold already) and serve. I suggest to be sure that your knife is wet when you cut as it will go much easier.

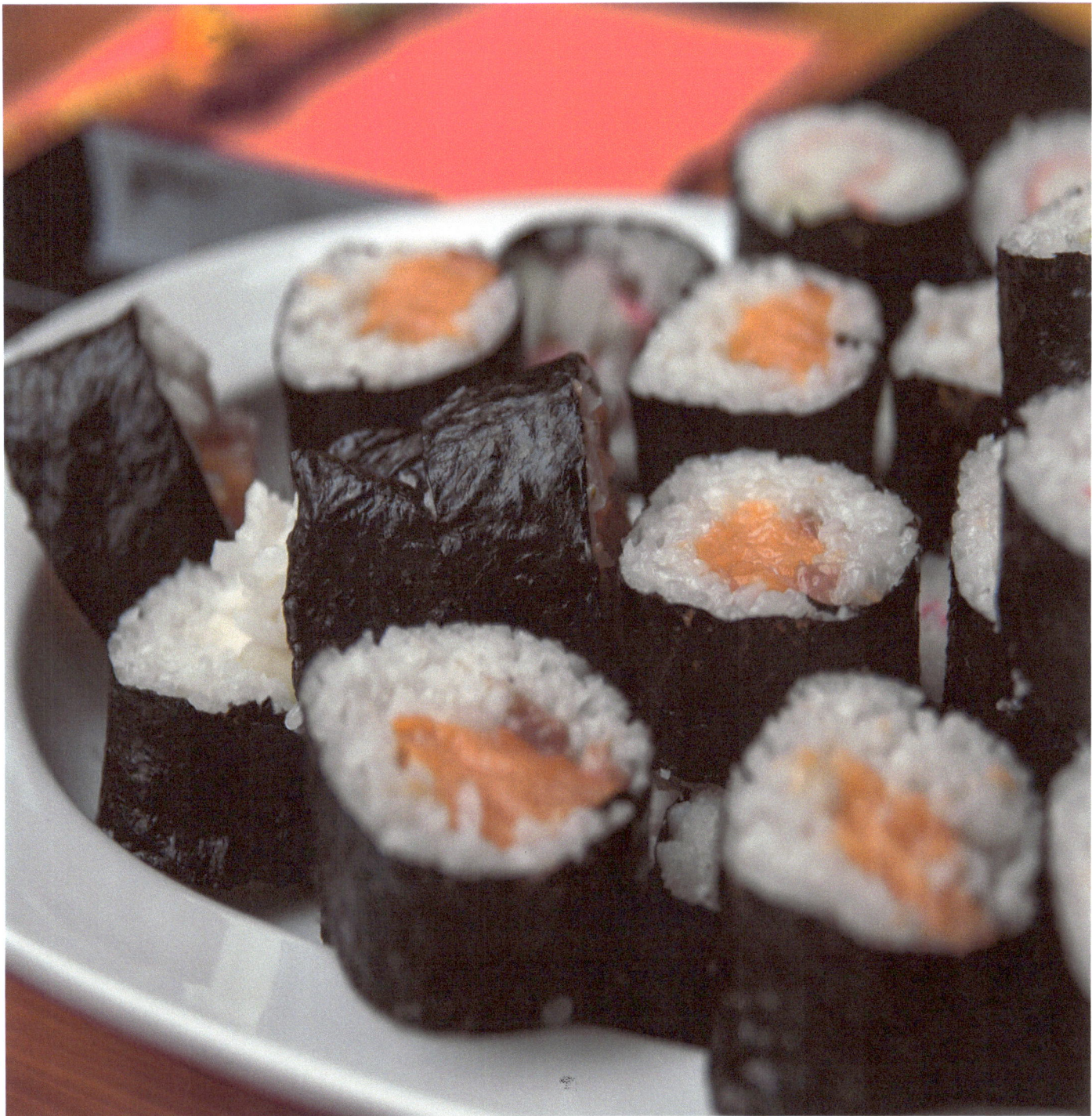

Cauliflower with egg and onion

You'll want to include cauliflower as one of the key vegetables you eat on a regular basis if you want to receive the fantastic health benefits provided by the cruciferous vegetable family. You can find several dozen studies linking cauliflower-containing diets to cancer prevention, particularly with respect to the following types of cancer: bladder cancer, breast cancer, colon cancer, prostate cancer, and ovarian cancer. This connection between cauliflower and cancer prevention should not be surprising, since cauliflower provides special nutrient support for three body systems that are closely connected with cancer development as well as cancer prevention. As with all vegetables be sure not to overcook cauliflower if you wish to even bother to cook it. Below we didn't cook it though we assume someone may not like it this way.

Ingredients:

- 1 cauliflower
- 1 big onion
- 2 eggs
- olive oil

Method:

Cut cauliflower florets into small pieces since you are going to boil it. Prepare pan heat oil and bring nicely chopped onion to brown colour. Then add cauliflower and keep stirring until its a bit softer than normally. Add in eggs and stir until eggs are done. Serve after you use salt and a pinch of pepper to taste.

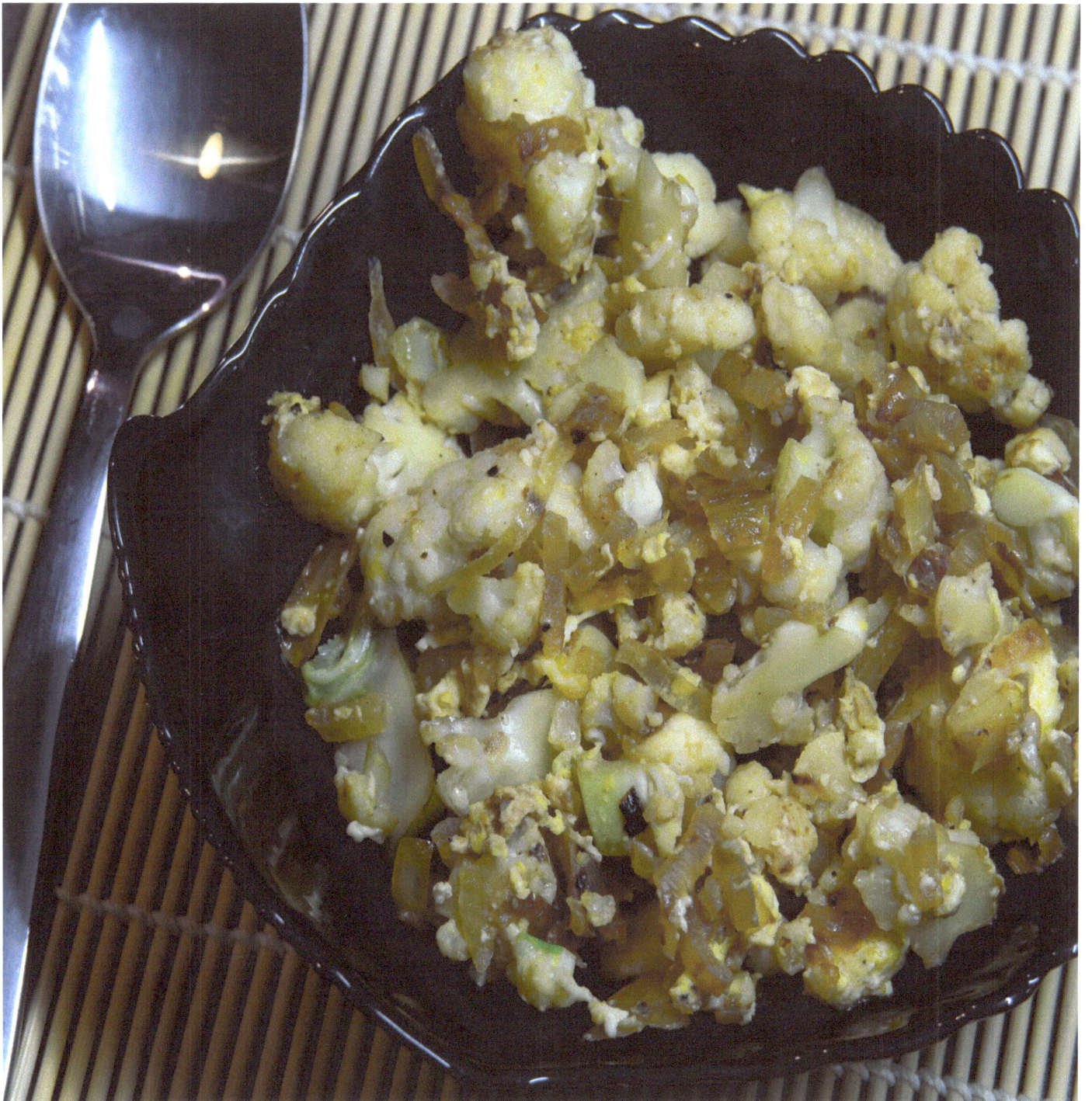

Mussels on wine and garlic

Mussels are a widely available seafood with many health benefits. Mussels are a high protein food source. Their low fat content makes them potentially healthier than other protein sources, such as beef, which can contain a lot of saturated fat.

Cautions About Mussels

Mussels are prone to the same types of bacterial contamination as other seafood and should only be prepared if they are live, as dead mussels quickly deteriorate. Mussels which are dead will be slightly open and will not close when disturbed. Mussels are a healthy and nutritious addition to most meals and can provide real benefits to health and well being. They are low in fat and high in nutrients like omega-3 and iron, and are also delicious and versatile. Careful preparation and monitoring health warnings about fishing areas will ensure that both commercial and self-harvested mussels are safe to eat and enjoy.

Ingredients:

- garlic (3-4 cloves) - chopped
- onion (1 piece of a decent size)
- mussels (depends but roughly 1kg is enough for dinner for two)
- herbs such as parsley or spring onion (optional)

Method:

Heat pot with a bit of oil, put in chopped garlic and sliced onion and stir fry for 1-2 minutes. Add mussels (that you have washed them first and put aside) and continue to stir the mixture. Here either add a glass of wine or a cup of water to the mixture. Once heated again add salt and pepper to taste. You may as well add a pinch of mix herbs. Bring it to boil and serve when mussels are cooked (open). Side dish is up to you, in France common side dish is fries, surprise! or bread.

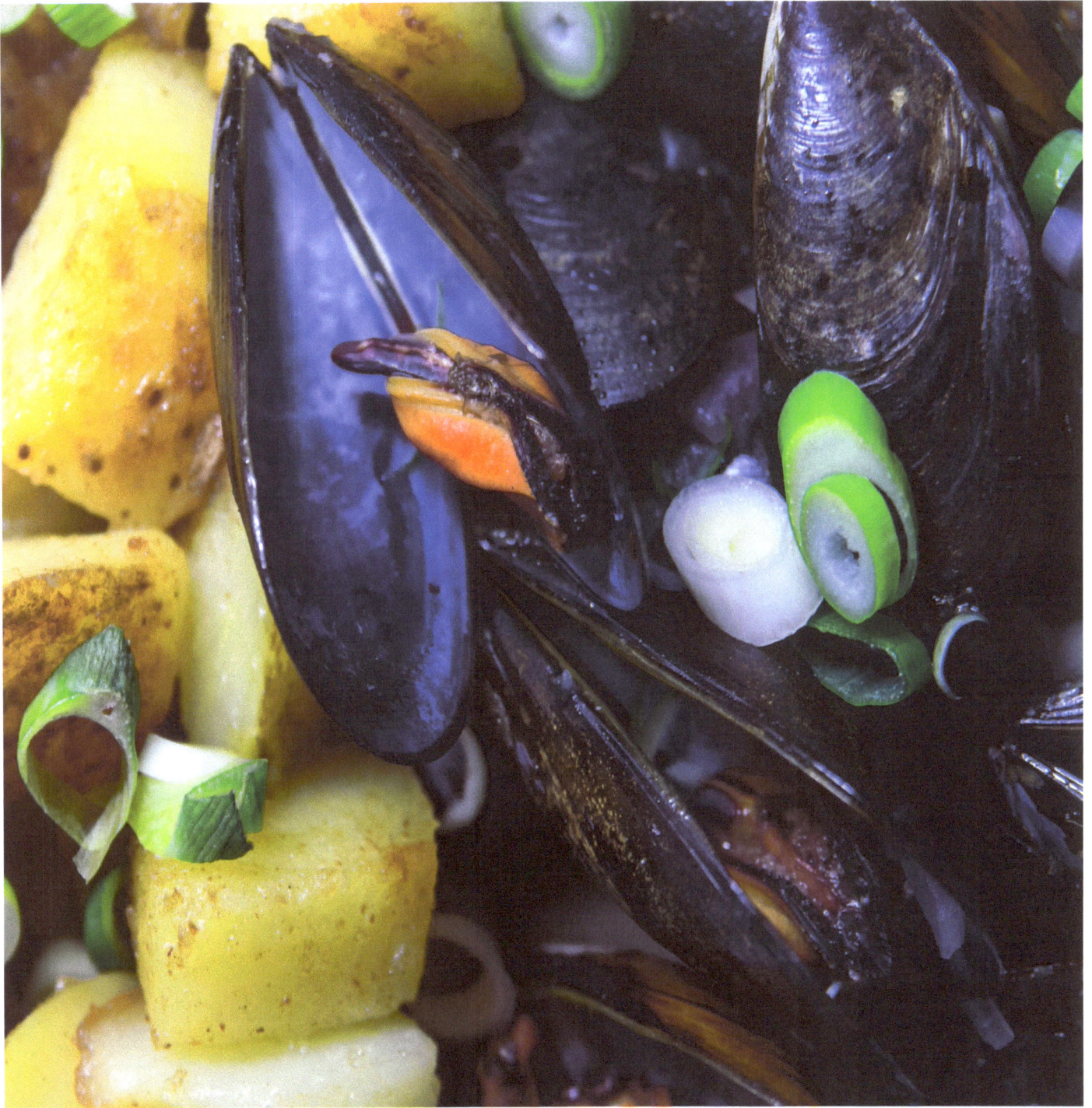

Grill chicken drumstick with mashed potatoes

Have you end up 'only' with chicken drumsticks, leftover of green vegetable, and potato... has no idea what to cook for your today's lunch? Just grill chicken drumsticks in the oven and serve over mashed potatoes. Sounds great to us. This is a quick meal to fix, and it's easy on the budget. What is going to take you the most time is to grill the chicken so make sure to start with that.

Ingredients:

- chicken drumstick
- potatoes
- butter
- milk
- green vegetable such as broccoli

Method:

Heat up oven up till 200°C degree and wash the chicken drumsticks. Put the chicken into the heated oven for about 30 minutes until chicken is done. You will see by crispy skin or you may try by poking into the meat. If tender then it is done. Peel and cut potatoes into pieces where smaller pieces ensure that you will have it boiled faster. Boil potatoes till soft, then pour the excess water from the boiled potatoes. Add salt, butter and milk to the boiled potatoes and blend till it become mashed potatoes. Take a shower before grill chicken is ready and you can serve.

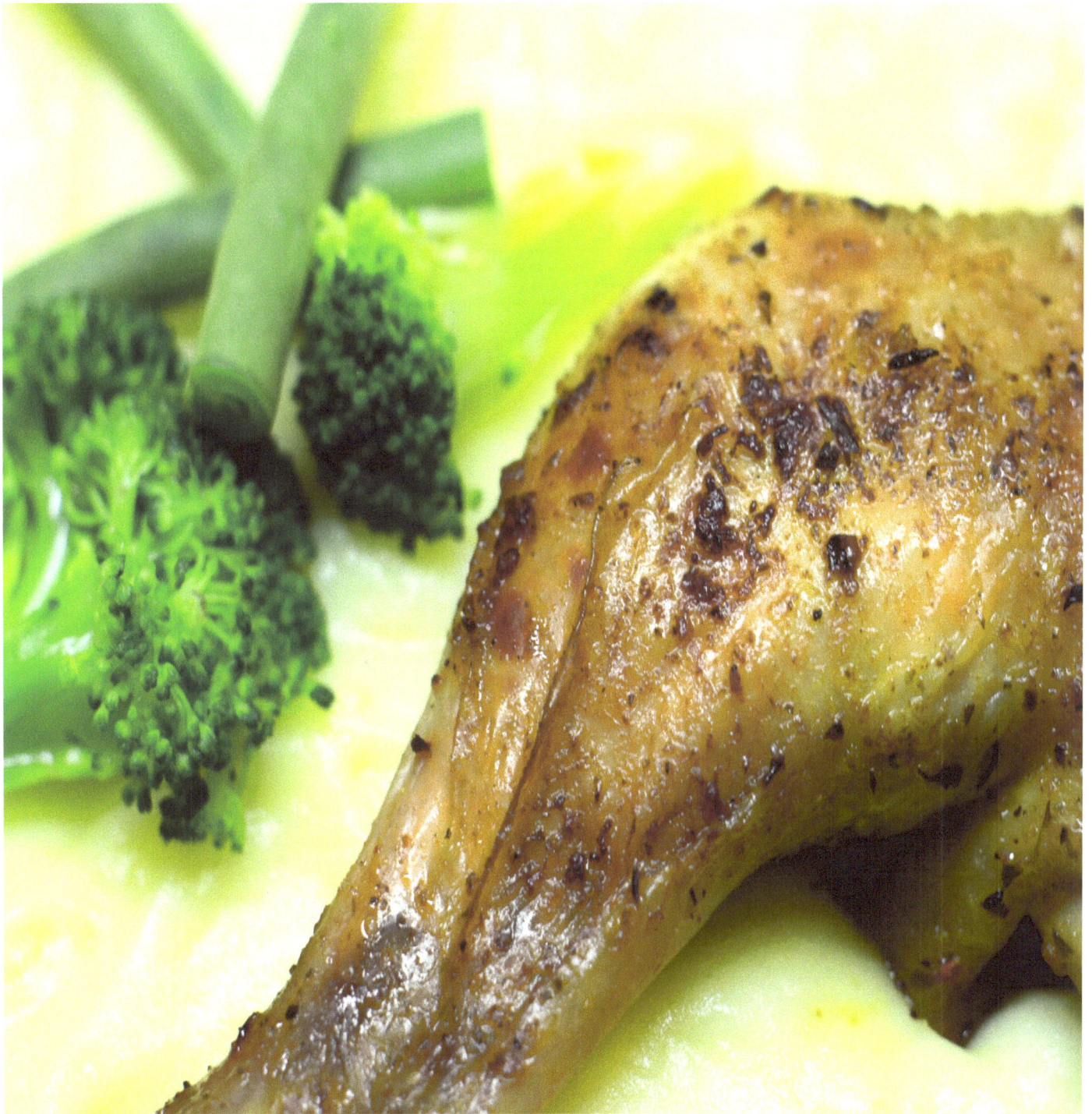

Minced meat with eggplant

You should consider this dish to be a candidate for 'cheat' day. Not that it would be unhealthy but for the sake of pork meat. Pork meat has nothing to do with healthy diet and we know that. Nevertheless following proverb 'do things in moderation', we believe that time by time one shall eat something more fatty

Ingredients:

- minced meat
- 1 egg plant
- sesame oil
- soya sauce
- dark soya sauce
- salt
- pepper
- oyster sauce

Method:

Marinate minced meat with sesame oil, soya sauce, salt and pinch of black pepper and set aside. Cut egg plant into reasonable pieces (not huge). Pour hot water into the cut egg plant to soften it for 3 minutes. Heat pan with oil and toss in minced meat. Continue to stir the minced meat so that it looks evenly done. Add in eggplant and stir mixture. Add dark soy sauce, soya sauce, salt and oyster sauce to taste. Add in 1/4 cup of water and continue to cook until the eggplant is softened enough. Serve warm.

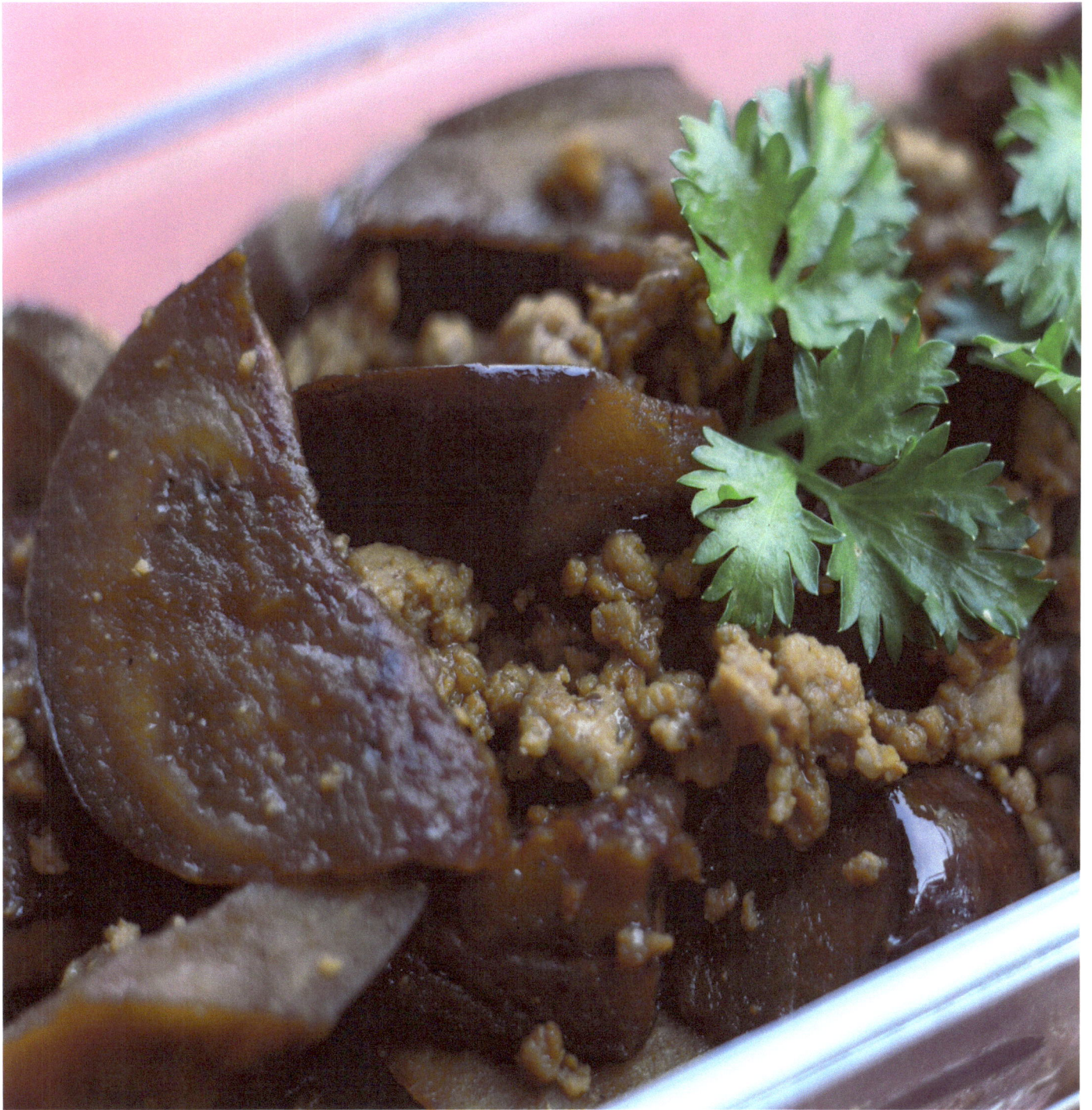

Chicken Porridge

Though endless versions of savory rice porridge (also known as congee) exist worldwide, we would show you this easy baseline you may wish to tune up the way you want. Feel free to add more garnishes like, green, soy sauce, fish sauce, fried shallots, or roasted salted peanuts to spice up this dish though it is tasty enough on itself.

Ingredients:

- jasmine rice (1/2 cup)
- chicken meat (to be sliced into pices and marinated with salt, soya sauce and pinch of salt)
- sesame oil
- soya sauce
- salt

Method:

Marinate jasmine rice with 1 tablespoon of sesame oil, 2 table spoons of soya sauce and 1 table spoon of salt. Set aside for a few minutes to extend the flavour. Add 3 and 1/2 cups of water into the marinated rice and cook with rice cooker if possible. Add chicken slices into the mixture as soon as it is boiling. Stir the mixture and add more water shall it be too thick. Let it cook and eventually (when cooker is turned off) add salt to taste and enjoy.

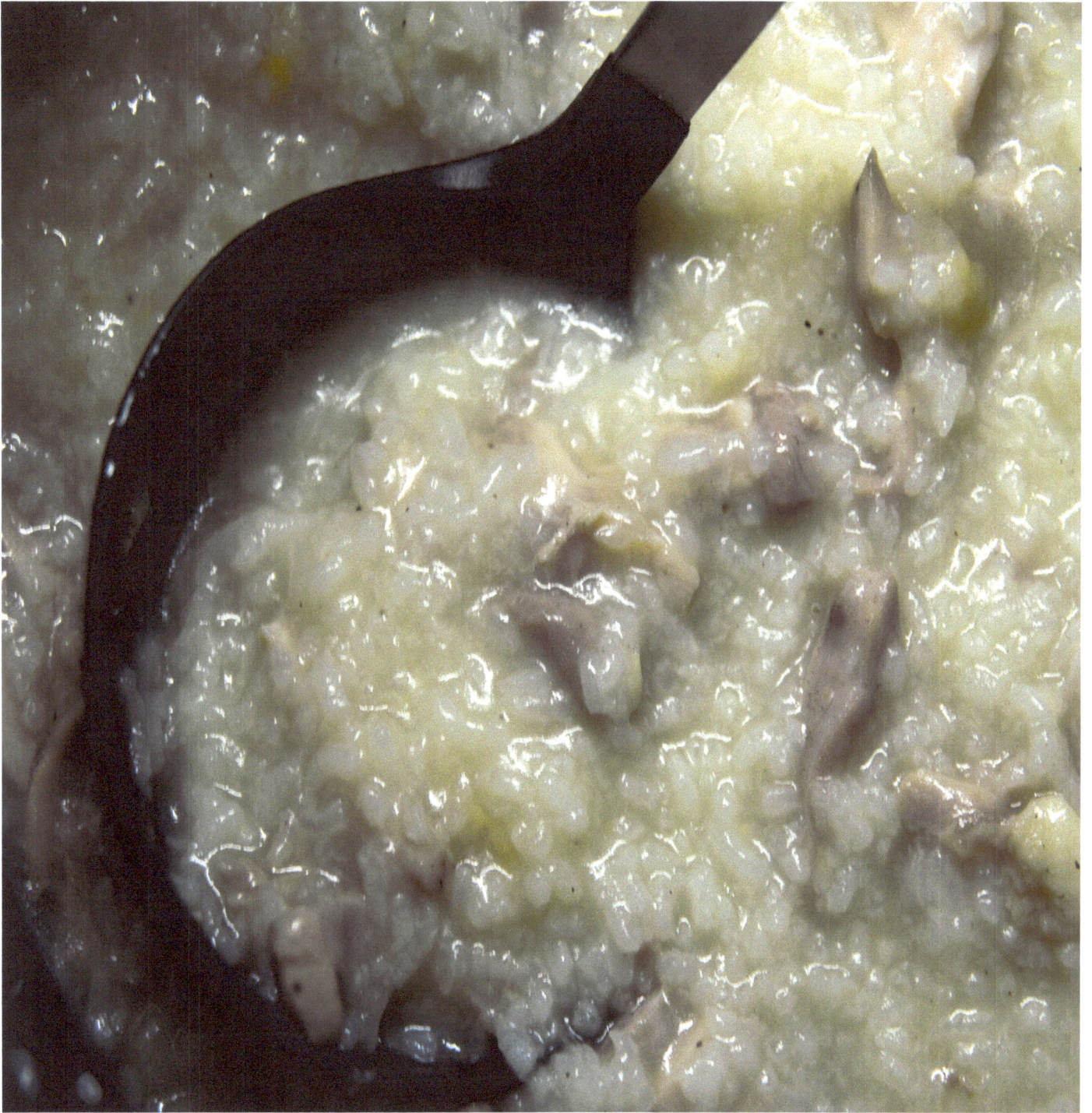

Cous-Cous with cheaty vegetable

This is quite a perfect summer meal. What I love about this recipe is the practicality: it is both quick to make and can wait for you; there's no hurry to serve. It's also a satisfying vegetarian meal (if you exclude sausage). We've included sausage this time since I was starving for something which has some meaty potential however it can be well excluded.

Ingredients:

- sausage
- 1 egg plant
- tomatoes
- soya sauce
- spinach
- salt
- pepper
- spring onion
- cous cous
- mushrooms

Method:

Firstly, prepare cous-cous which is likely just to be poured by boiling water with a bit of olive oil. Then, heat oil in large pot over medium-low heat. Place onion and cook, stirring occasionally, until onions begin to soften and turn translucent, about 4 minutes. Add in sausage and mushrooms and stir; cook another 2 minutes. Pour in the tomatoes, and if necessary some water to make gravy. Add in all other vegetables and bring to boil. When cous-cous has soaked all the water slowly pour the vege mixture into the cous-cous; stir. Cover pot immediately and remove from the heat. Let it stand, covered, for 5 minutes. Fluff cous-cous with a fork. The cous-cous should have absorbed about half of the cooking sauce. Serve at slightly warmer than room temperature.

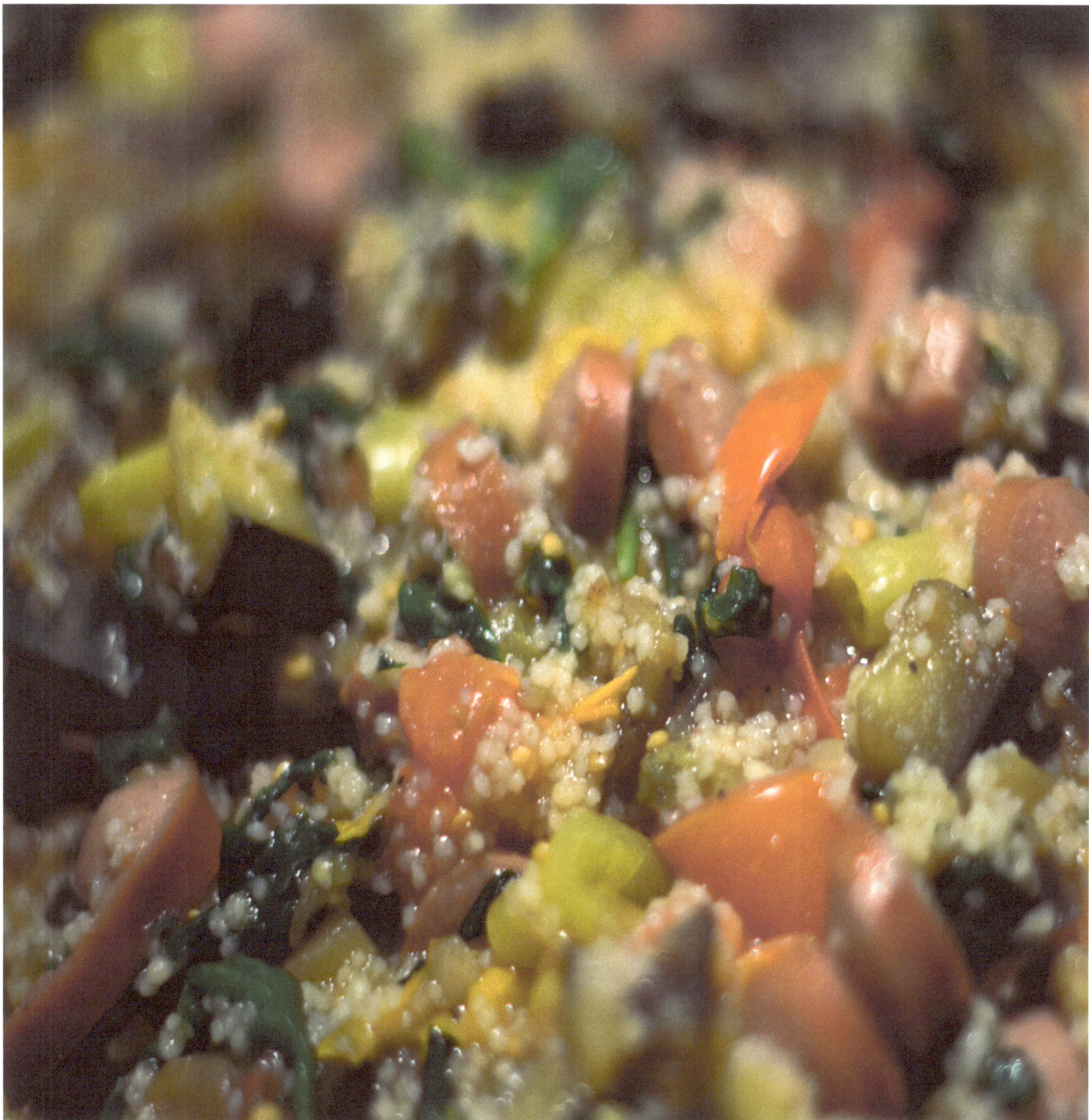

Grilled Trout with Rosemary

This simple presentation is a go-to summer recipe that allows the flavor of the fish to shine. Hand by hand with rosemary it is also extremely tasty - and convenient. A delicious trout meal can take under 15 minutes to prepare and cook. Research shows that trout and other oil rich fish can play a vital role in preventing deaths from heart disease- and yet most of us fail to eat enough to do us good. In addition to medical research into heart disease, there is growing evidence to demonstrate the importance of Omega-3 in brain and retina development in infants. Research indicated that people who obtained approximately 25 percent of their total caloric intake from lean protein sources like fish were more likely to lose weight, retain lean muscle mass and feel fuller after eating than people who received only 12 percent of their calories from protein. This was especially true when the high-protein intake was coupled with exercise and an overall decrease in daily calories.

So don't miss out - pick up a trout and head for a healthier lifestyle.

Ingredients:

- two trout fish
- one stalk of fresh rosemary
- salt
- potatoes
- broccoli
- cherry tomatoes
- mushrooms
- white sauce
- lemon

Method:

First work on fish. Clean it properly, and then just salt it, squeeze all over a lemon and garnish with rosemary. Shall you be concerned to have more impact with final taste you can sprinkle all over a bit of fish grill spice. Now put fish in pre-heated oven at least for 15 min. Now in meantime work on side dish. This is optional since it has nothing much to do with grilled trout. Boil potatoes, there is nothing to talk about. Aside heat oil in large pot over medium-low heat. Place onion and cook, stirring occasionally, until onions begin to soften and turn golden brown, about 4 minutes. Add in water, maximum half a litre, stir, and keep adding ingredients such as mushrooms; broccoli, put those not yet completely boiled potatoes and lastly cherry tomatoes. Keep stiring and turn off the heat and only then put in white sauce. Don't let it boil together with that. Let it stand, covered, for 5 minutes.

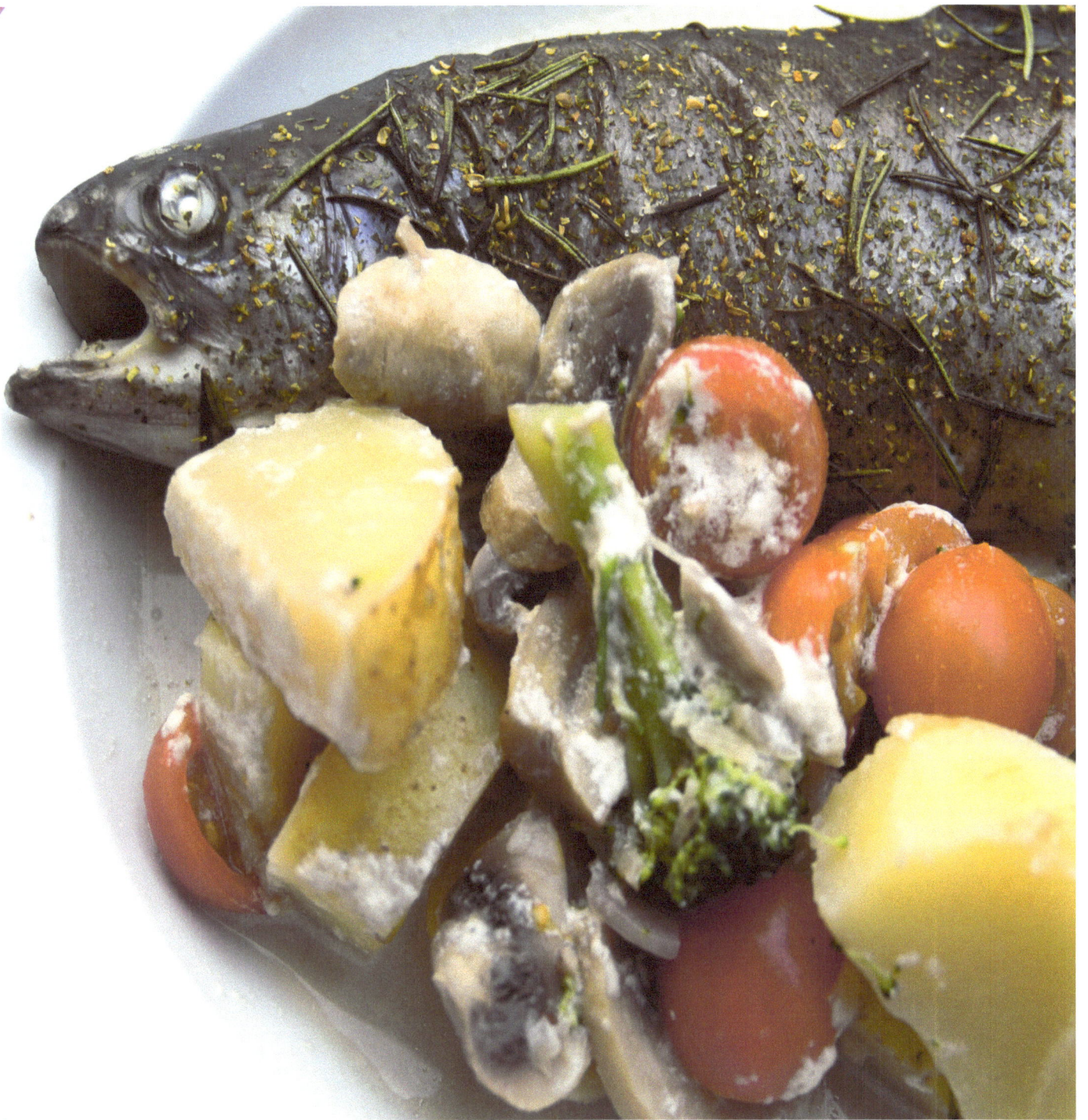

White Broccoli

Usually don't give this to your husband unless he asks for it. Not that its not nice but more that it can be seen as penurious. For those who likes something more sweet, just use apples instead of broccoli. Apple confronting yogurt tend to release its sweetness.

Ingredients:

- broccoli
- white yogurt

Method:

This is indeed simple. Steam broccoli while keeping that nice lush green colour or just put it on bowl and pour hot water all over. After few minutes get rid of the water and serve with zero fat white yogurt as a dip. Simple as that though surprisingly satisfying.

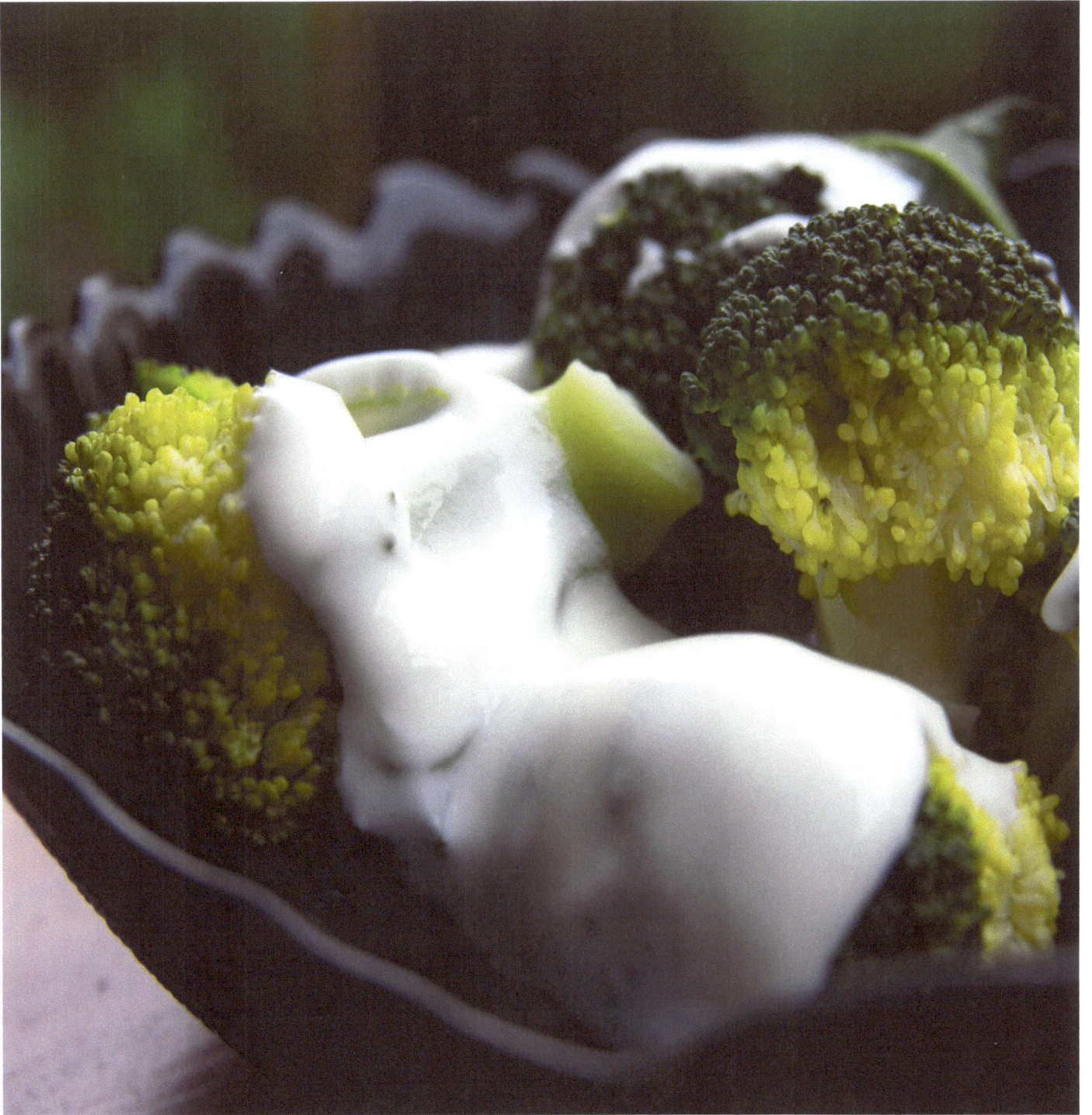

Natural prawns with egg coat

Whether you claim you like sea food you ought to love prawns. And not only that since facts supports us to eat more! Because of their many nutritional benefits, prawns are considered by a variety of health experts to be among the healthiest foods in the world. Prawns are a great source of high quality protein, and provide some of the most important vitamins and minerals that make up a healthy diet. They are surprisingly low in calories and are made up of extremely healthy cholesterol.

Ingredients:

- fresh prawns
- 2 eggs
- olive oil

Method:

Don't spoil natural taste of prawns. Be careful to not overfry prawns as they may become hard, chewy and a bit dry. Stir fry prawns on olive oil for few minutes on medium heat. Just before you think they may be done put a bit of white wine and eggs. Keep stirring until eggs are done. Towards the end put salt and you may serve. The tougest part on this dish is actually to get fresh prawns at least in central Europe.

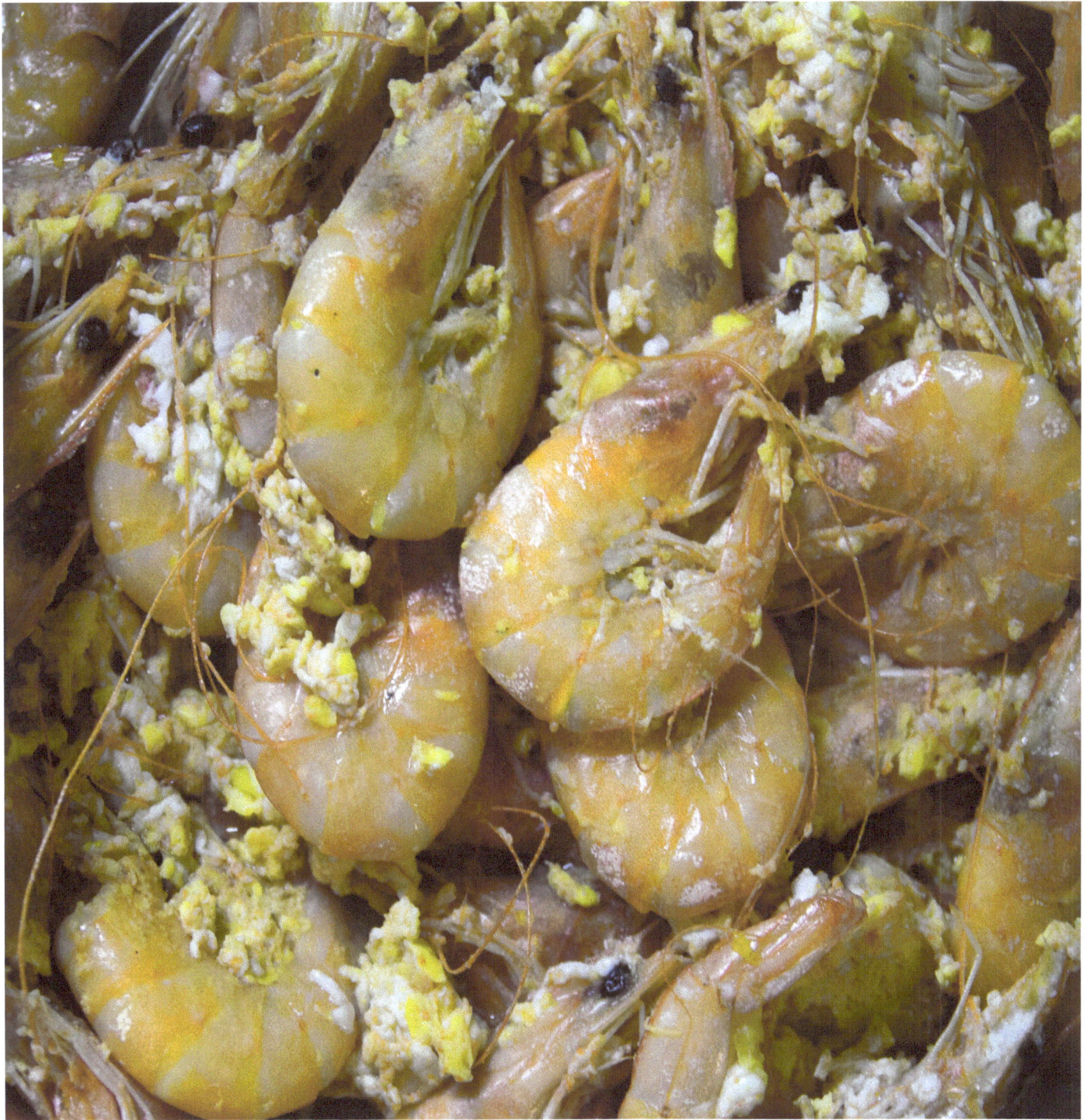

Classic Eggless Past (Spaghetti)

This underestimated dish is supposed to be only for novice cook. You may know the joke that someone is that bad cook who is not even able to cook spaghetti. Well, yes indeed it is easy... and that's why we have it here! This is the only pasta dish in the whole book since you should avoid eating pasta whenever you want to be on diet.

Ingredients:

- 250g of bio eggless spaghetti
- tomatoes
- tomato puree
- parmesan cheese
- olive oil
- fresh basil or chives
- garlic

Method:

Bring a large pan of salted water to the boil, add the spaghetti and cook according to the packet instructions.
Meanwhile set a large frying pan over medium heat and when hot, tip in the oil and then chopped onion. Cook for 5 mins until starting to soften, stirring occasionally. Add the garlic, cook 2 mins more until the onions start to turn golden. When the onion has softened, pour at least a glass of water and tip in cuts of tomatoes and half the basil. Add tomato puree too to achieve darker red colour and richer consistence. Leave to gently bubble for 15 mins until the sauce has thickened and looks pulpy. Stir occasionally and break up any large clumps of tomato with the back of your spoon.

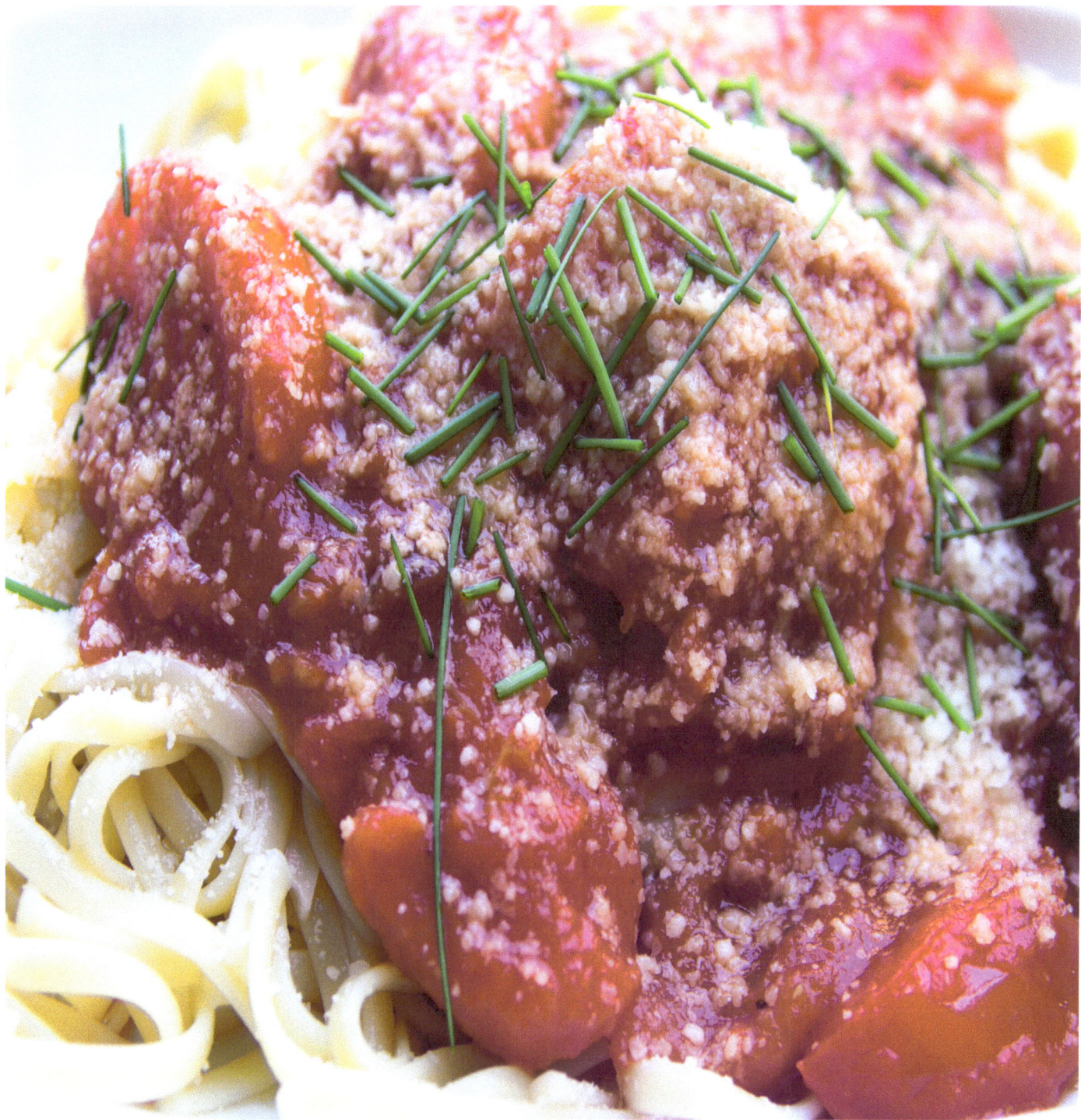

Salads

Salads... this is a huge topic and theoretically you can combine almost all possible vegetables, seeds, or for meat eaters as well some light meat such as fish or chicken. These few salads we show here are just fragment of what you can dare to think of. So release your potential and go creative!

Vegetable salad with mandarin orange

Let's witness that vegetable salat can be tasty without using any dressing. This tossed green salad with few not really usual ingredients simply sparkles with a marvelous mandarin orange juice. It will do a perfect light dinner.

Ingredients:

- 1 big cucumber
- 3 tomatoes
- 2 red pepper
- handful of sunflower seeds
- mozzarella cheese
- green veggie such as baby spinach will do or like us here we use 'Eruca sativa'
- 1 canned mandarin

Method:

Cut all ingredients no matter in what order and pour them all into one big bowl so that you can easily mix them. Put few drops of virgin olive oil and a pinch of salt together with all sunflower seeds that you have. Mix properly and let it cool down for the vegetable to absorb that salt. To have richer taste, do not put the salad back into the fridge before it is being served.

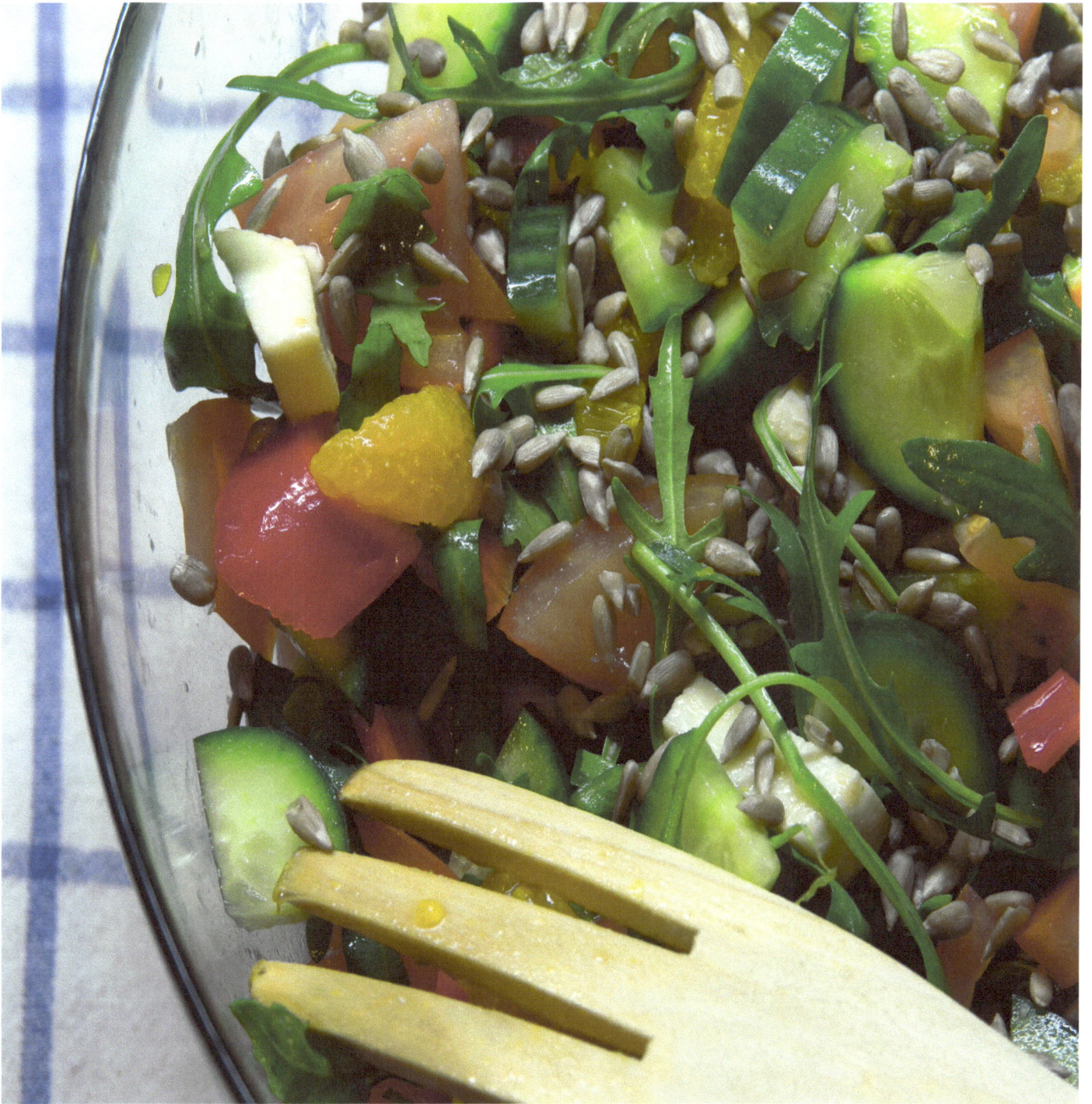

Vegetable salad with fried shallots

Fried shallots add sweetness and a crouton-like crunch to this simple chinese style green salad which can be used as side dish for main or even such as light dinner. You can go creative and use practically any lettuce.

Ingredients:

- ice lettuce
- shallots - to be cut into thin slices
- soy sauce
- oyster sauce

Method:

Pour hot water over ice lettuce and leave it for few minutes, or until it reaches your desirable texture. Pour out hot water and let it drain so that it will not have excess water later on. Heat the pan with oil, and pan fry shallots/onions until it reaches golden brown. Mix the drained ice lettuce with soy sauce, oyster sauce and leftover oil from previously pan frying shallots. Toss fried shallots on top of the salad and serve.

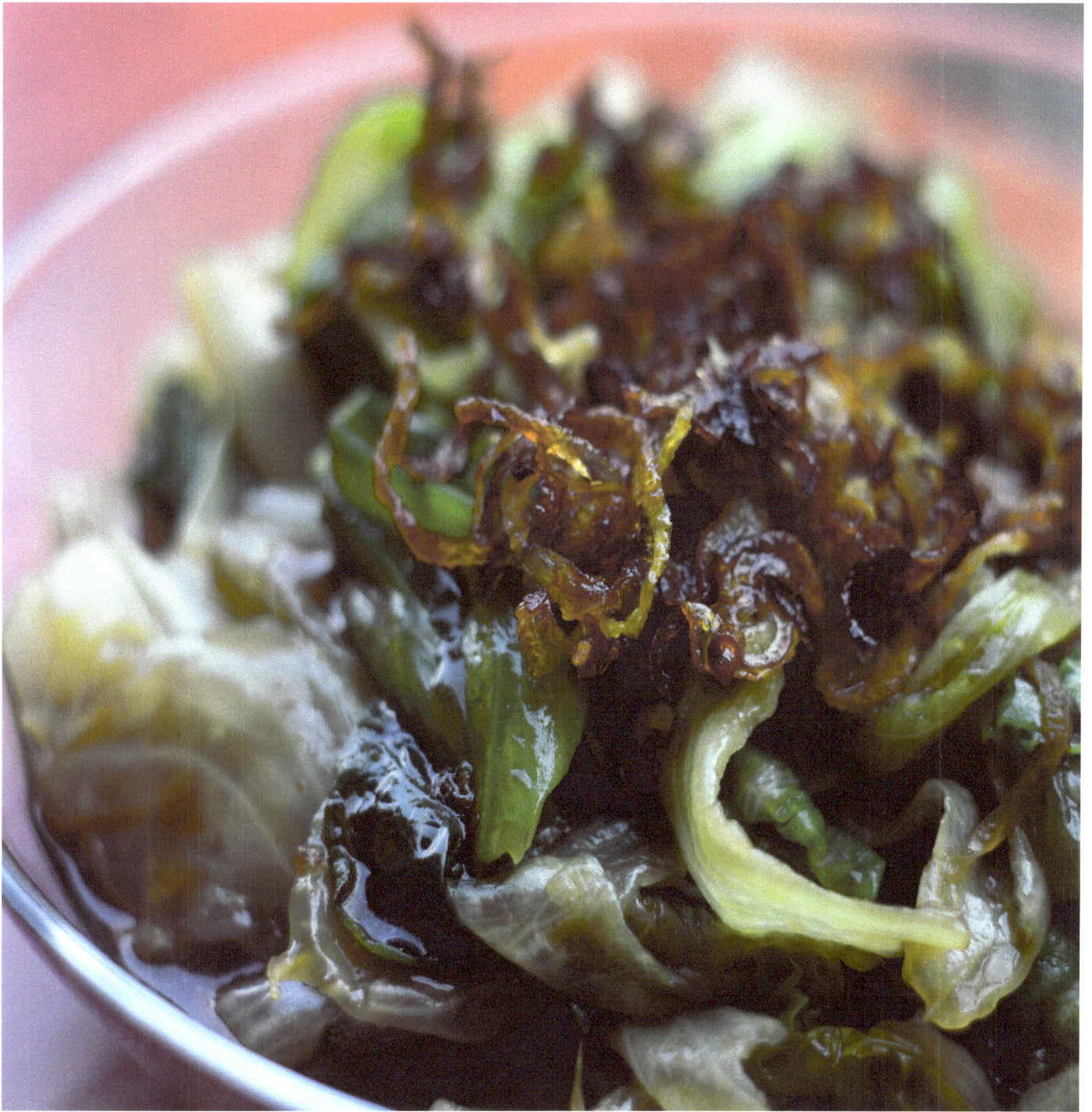

Cucumber sour salad

Around summer we start having cucumber salads almost every night with dinner as the cucumbers are growing a bit out of control in the garde or climbing up the tomato cages. Every weekend my parents bring in a handful, so we peel them and chop them up for a simple salad consisting of nothing more than the cucumbers, some vinegar, pepper, salt and sugar. If you have mix in dill or basil but true is you don't really need the herbs; cucumbers are crunchy and cool with just some vinegar, salt and pepper.

Ingredients:

- cucumber
- pinch of pepper, salt, sugar

Method:

Shred cucumber after washing it or if you prefer without skin on grater. Prepare mix aside in cup, usually I use the one of 300 ml. There mix spoon of salt, sugar and vinegar. Fill with watter, then put pepper and mix until salt and sugar dissolve. Pour dressing over and you are done.

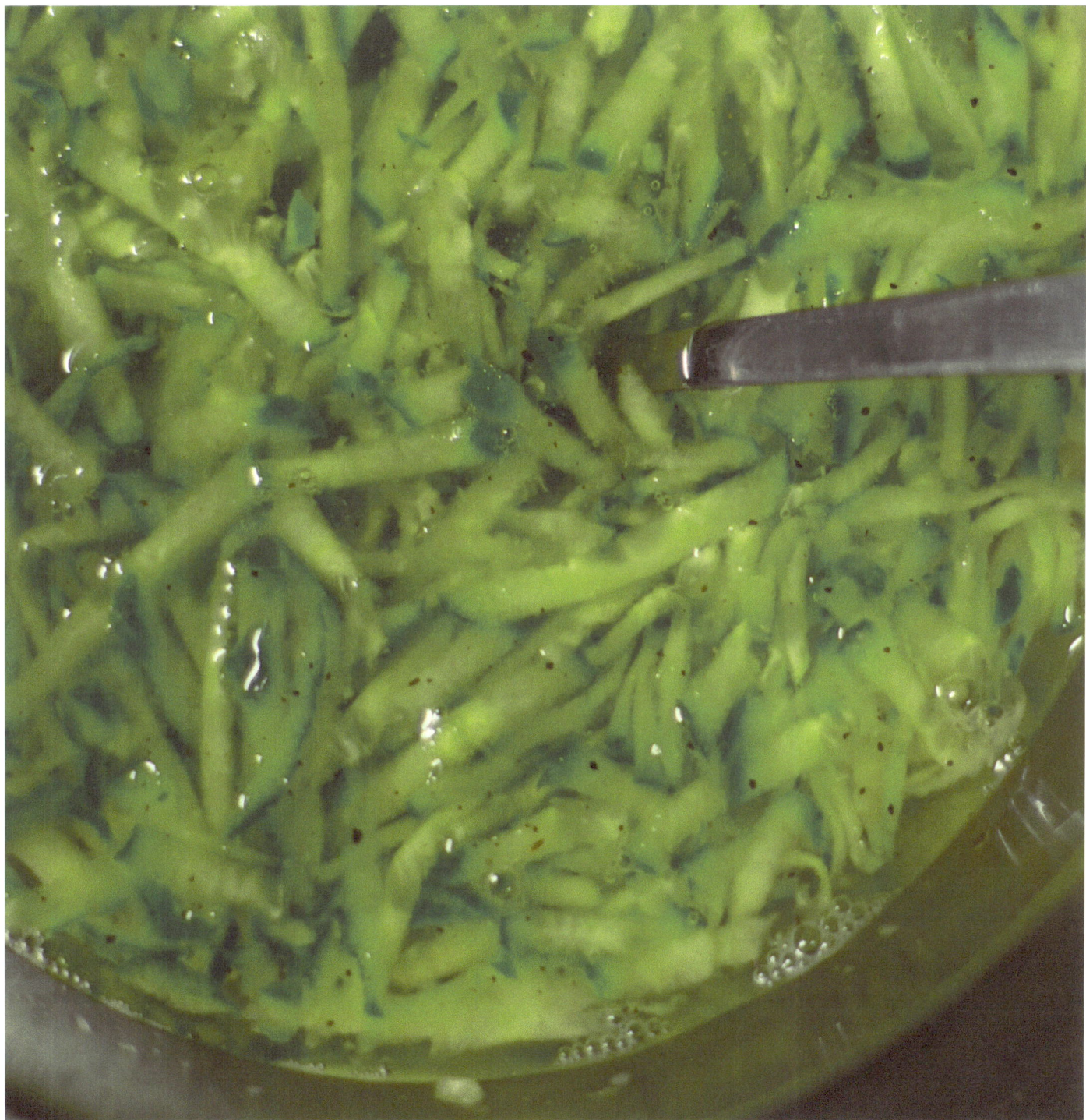

Vegetable salad with walnuts

Magic of this salat is hidden in walnuts. Walnuts not only taste great but are a rich source of heart-healthy monounsaturated fats and an excellent source of those hard to find omega-3 fatty acids. Like most nuts, they can easily be added to your Healthiest Way of Eating. Just chop and add to your favorite salad, vegetable dish, fruit, or dessert. Oh and don't peel them! Skin is the source of 90% of the whole vitamins.

Ingredients:

- cherry tomatoes
- ice lettuce
- cucumber
- cheese (balcanic or mozzarella)
- fresh spinach leaves
- parsley

Method:

This actually has no method since it is about to cut all put it on bowl and mix properly. What I suggest is to not put it back to fridge since flavour is richer when it is not too cold. Did I mention you are expected to unshell the nuts?

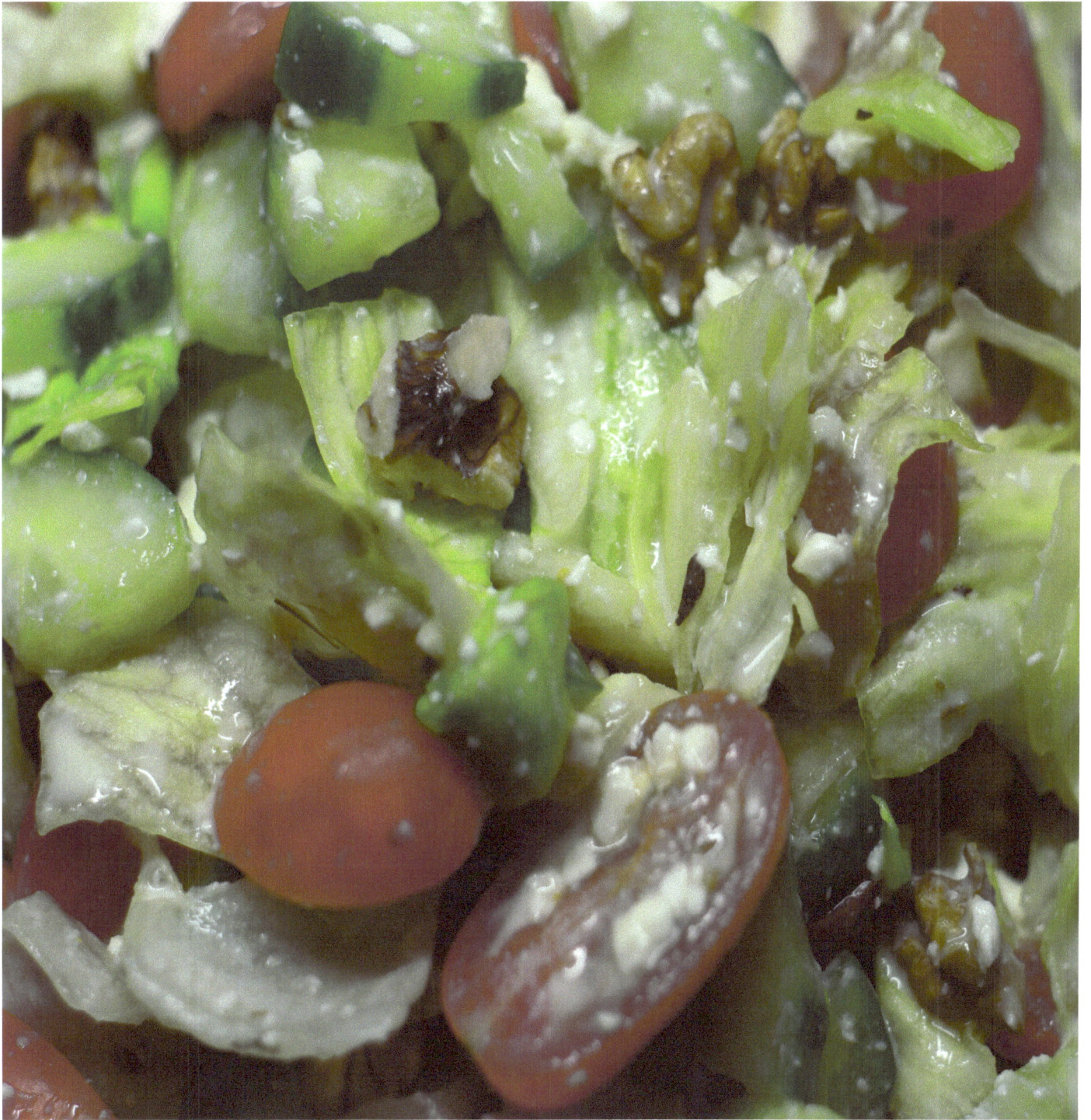

Soups

Soups are often serve alongside the meal. Sometimes you can use them as main dish but generally it is not common. They offer a heathly, low-fat flavoursome choice that provide the palette with tastes and textures that complement or contrast with the main dish. Following the nature of our book majority of our soups in our book are vegetarian. All of our soups are ideal as a light lunch or supper, and we believe there is something to please everyone.

Pea soup

This is not traditional version but the one we like the most. It's a delicious and healthy soup made from an impossibly short list of ingredients. No ham in this version, simply green peas and onions cooked until tender, then partially pureed. The vibrant green soup is finished with a gentle touch of fresh parsley to give the soup some more of a green depth. Keep in mind that fresh peas are uncomparable tastier than frozen one. If you need to use frozen, choose some 'brandy' one, not the cheapest in your favorite grocery store.

Ingredients:

- package of fresh peas, some 250g (or use frozen one when you don't have another choice)
- 2 eggs
- parsley
- white cream (sour - healtier but sweet is tastier though, make your choice)
- 1 onion
- vegetable stock (better version is home made, but vegetable stock cube will do)

Method:

Cut onion, don't bother with shape or size, stir fry till golden colour with a bit of oil. Add vegetable stock and a bit of water. Heat for a while and add peas. Lct it simmer and boil two eggs in another pot. Once tender, blend peas and onion with mixer but not untill too fine. Serve in a bowl, covered with white cream, fresh parsley and nicely decorated eggs.

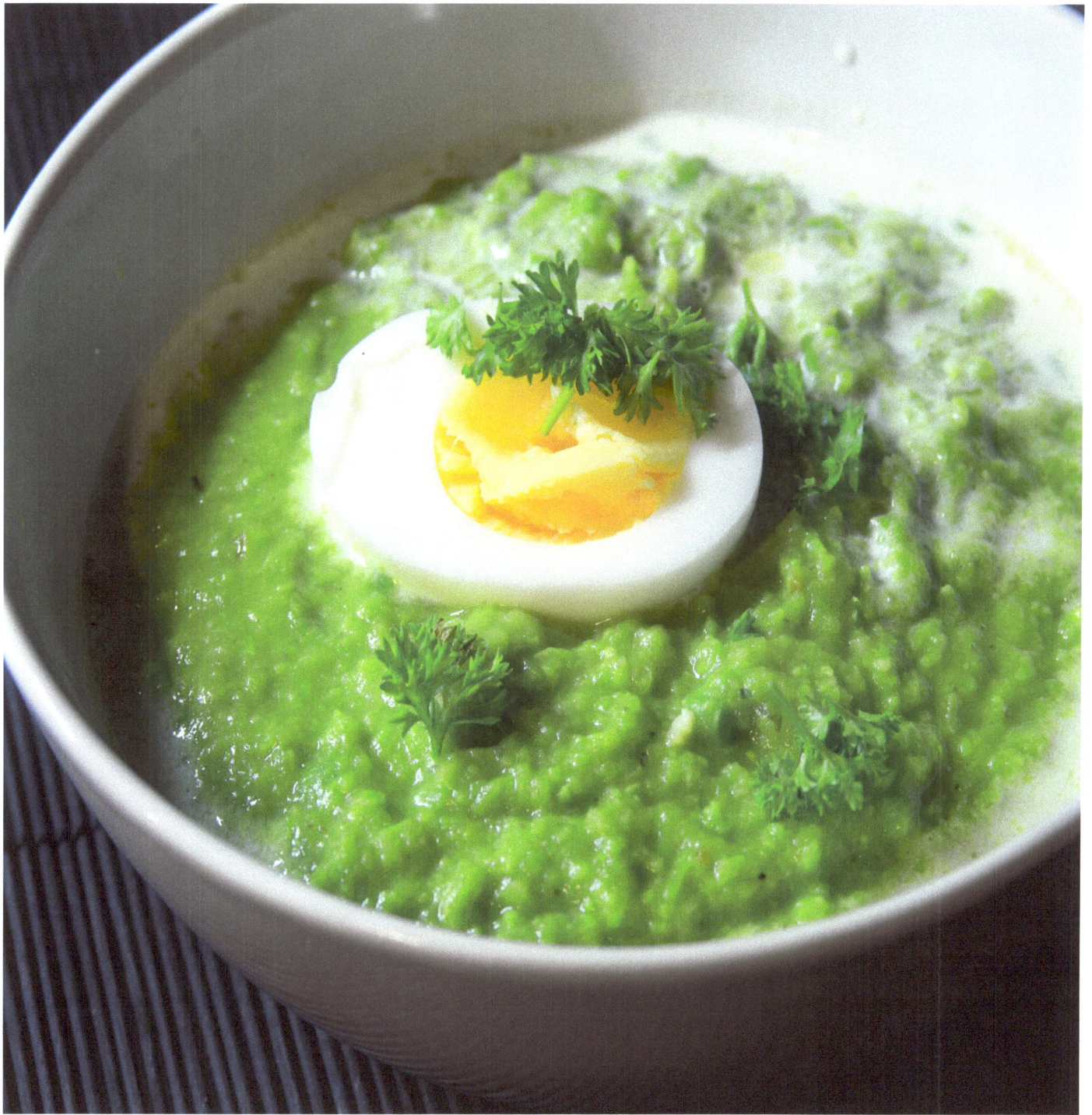

Hearty chicken and vegetable soup

This is pretty close to what my parents used to make. I've always thought of it as healthy and filling. There is no meat and very little fat in this recipe. I created this recipe on a cold and rainy winter day on which it definitely hit the spot.

Ingredients:

- 1/2 of chicken
- carrots
- spinach
- beetroot
- potatoes
- onion
- parsnip

Method:

First you will prepare chicken stock. You are lucky one if you have a pressure cooker. If so just put chicken into it for at least half an hour with salt. While this is cooking cut all the vegetables you will put in later. Cut it and prepare it the way that later you will be able to add into the pot based on how hard each and single vegetable is. Start with the onion, fry the onion until just before gold colour, and after that pour in all the stock from pressure cooker. Now keep adding vegetable, so hardest comes in first, so put potatoes, after a while carrots, parsnip, beetroot and last green, spinach or any other green you have. Cook until it reach your desirable softness. Serve immediately and enjoy this hearty soup.

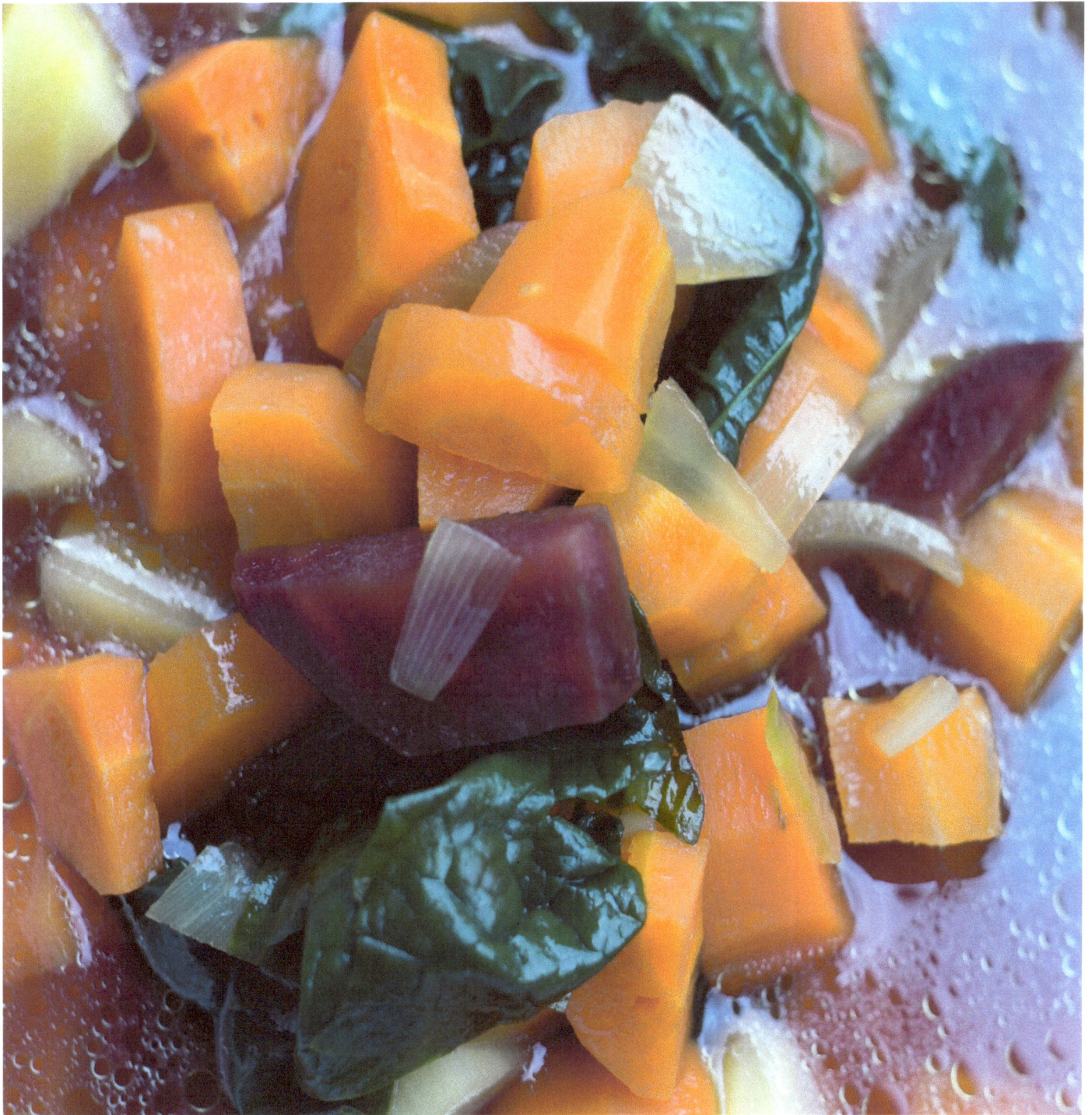

Sour pickled vegetable and tofu soup

This soup has just a hint of bitterness that is well balanced with the sour pickled mustard. As the soup simmers, the bitterness gets less prominent and other flavors blend in.

Ingredients:

- 150g of pickled vegetable (sour pickled mustard)
- 1 block of tofu
- 1 tomato
- 3 slices of ginger
- chicken stock

Method:

Boil chicken stock and cut vegee into slices. Put the sour vege first together with ginger, later add tofu and lastly tomato since it is the most soft ingredient. Boil low and after a few minutes turn it off. Notice that this soup requires completely no salt.

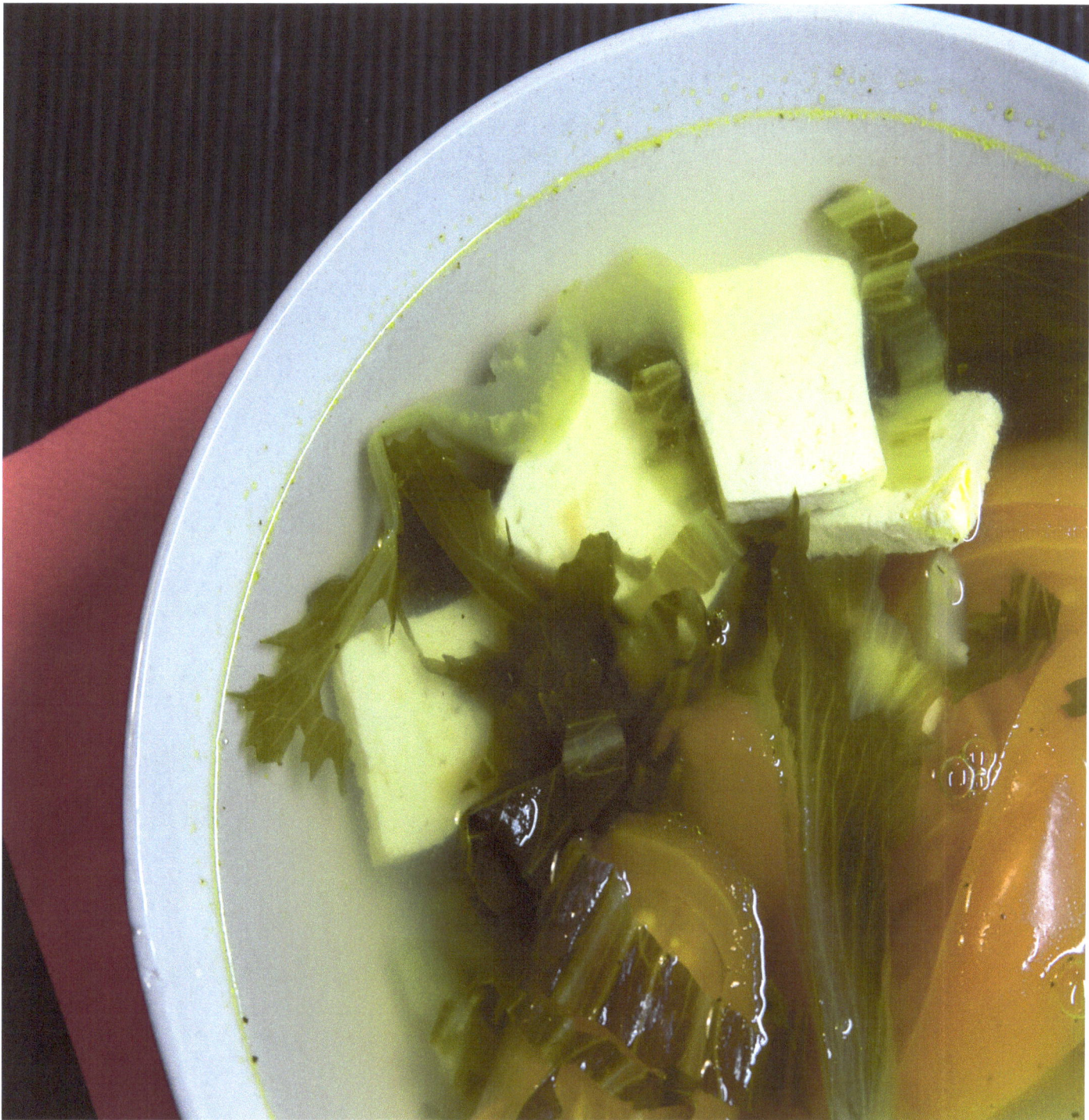

Spinach and egg soup

A very traditional egg drop soup with spinach, super simple and healthy. Adding a few drops of sesame oil adds a fragrant smell. Make sure you have fresh spinach leaves and if possible try with home-produced chicken eggs for richer flavor and colour

Spinach itself is low in saturated fat, and very low in cholesterol. It is also a good source of Niacin and Zinc, and a very good source of dietary fiber, Protein, Vitamin A, Vitamin C, Vitamin E (Alpha Tocopherol), Vitamin K, Thiamin, Riboflavin, Vitamin B6, Folate, Calcium, Iron, Magnesium, Phosphorus, Potassium, Copper and Manganese.

Ingredients:

- fresh spinach leaves
- 2 eggs
- fish stock or chicken stock (cube stock or preferably rich home made broth)

Method:

Heat the stock or just simply put your cube stock into the water. Once it is boiling add spinach leaves and salt to taste. Blend eggs in separate bowl up to united colour mixture and add them into the boiling mixture. Stir well and serve immediately.

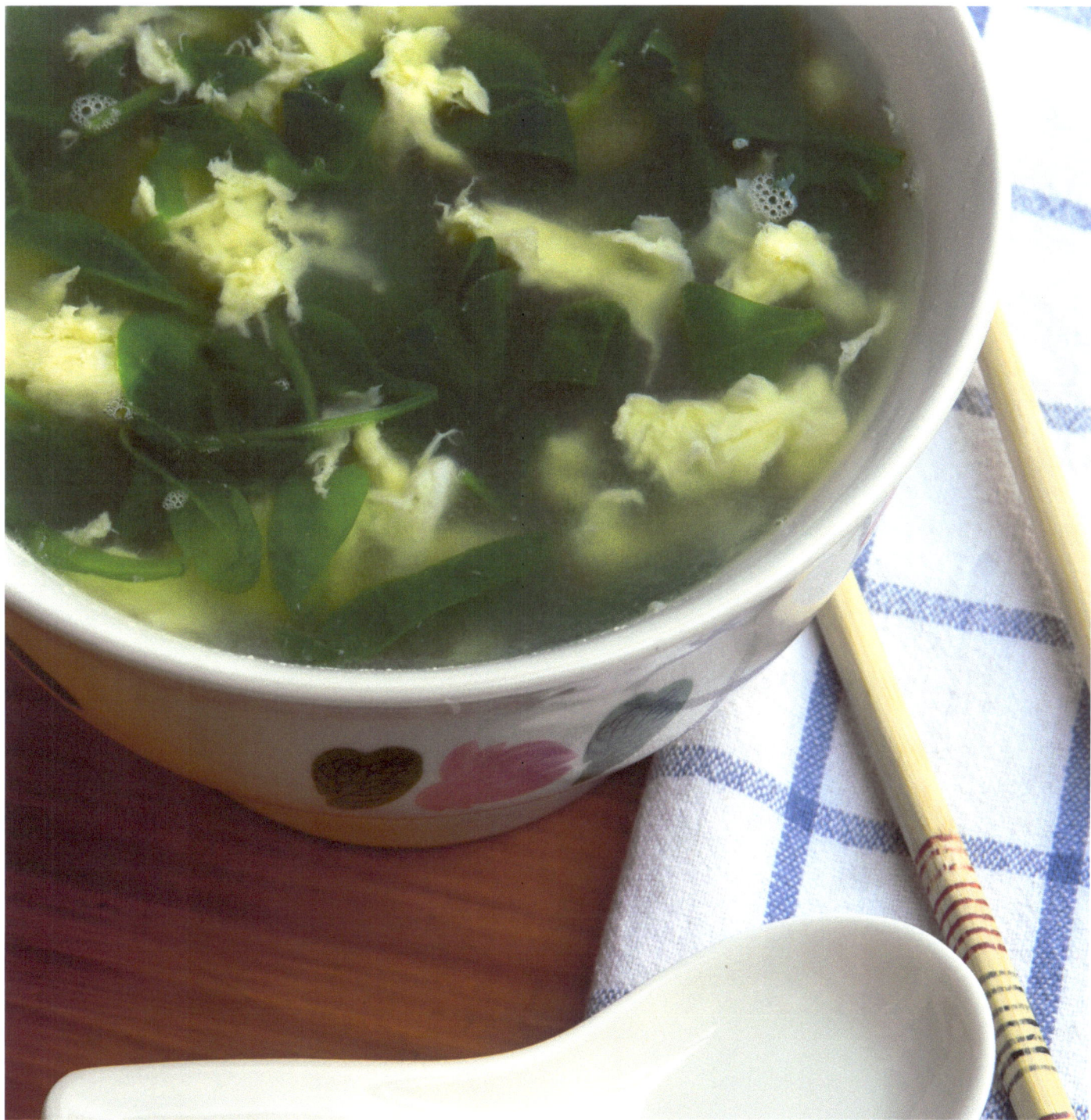

Garden Vegetable soup

Make an economical and wholesome meal from a simple vegetable soup with our easy, warming recipe. With this soup you can let your imagination to fly and let literary add any vege you can think of. So consider this recipe as just showing you the direction and modify as you wish.

Ingredients:

- 2 carrots
- fresh parsley
- 1 large onion
- 2 cloves of garlic
- quarter of cauliflower
- quarter of celery
- 1 white raddish
- a piece of broccoli
- half of the beetroot
- chicken stock (cube stock or preferably rich home made broth)

Method:

First cut everything into resonable pieces. Hear the pot with a bit of oil and add onion. Once onion is turning brown add the stock or just simply put your cube stock into the water. Once it is boiling add all the other ingredients and salt to taste. Boil until desired hardness is achieved - someone likes it tender we prefer harder so in our case we basically stop cooking just after few minutes. Garnish with chopped fresh parsley and serve with a piece of fresh bread.

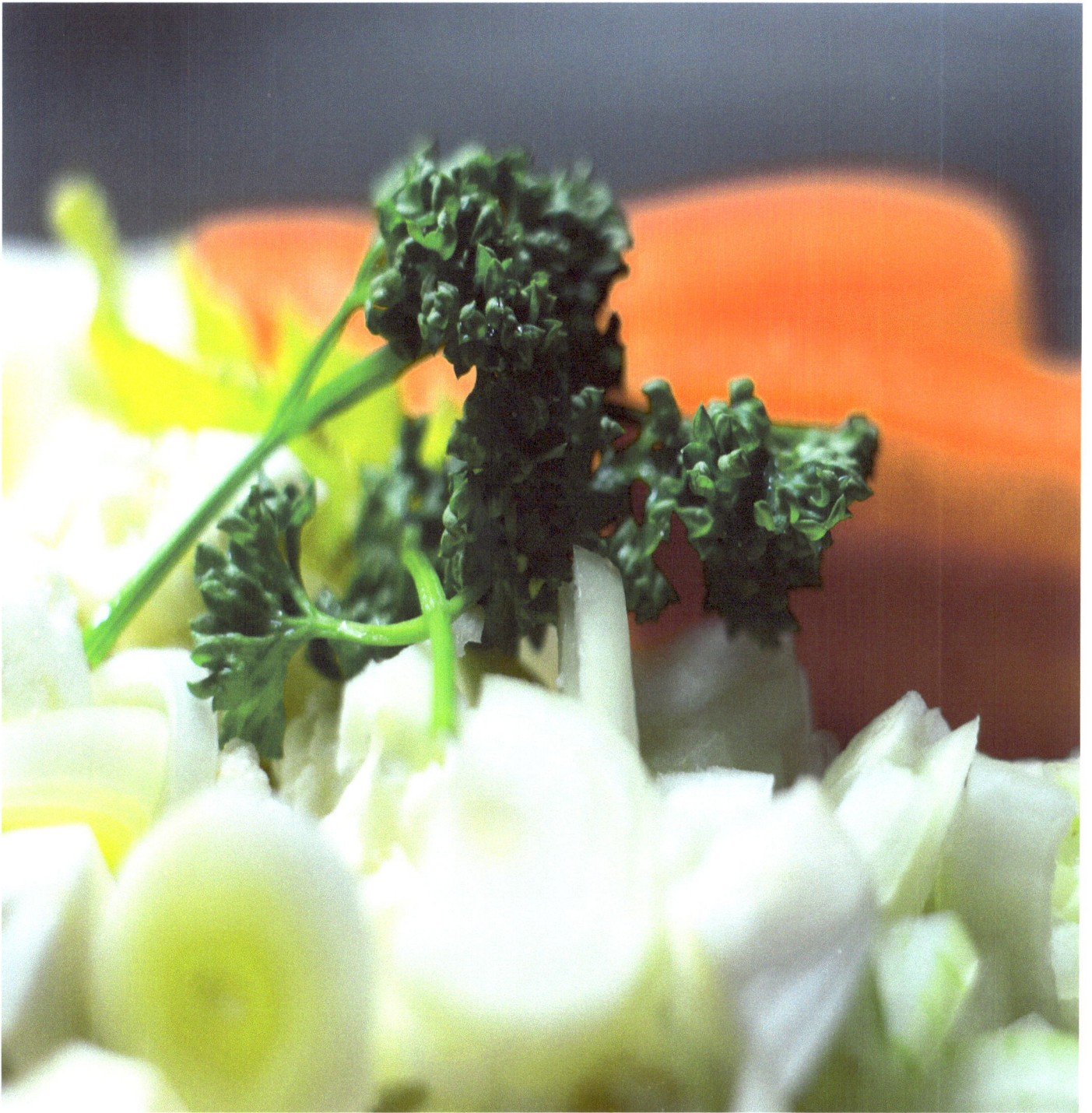

Broccoli soup

A smooth blended vegetable soup is on the table in less than twenty minutes. You can improve this simple recipe by adding an egg or serve it with buttered bread for example.

Ingredients:

- 1 broccoli
- spinach (fresh if possible)
- white cream for cooking

Method:

First cut broccoli into some small pieces or tear it down to its basic heads. Let it boil with maximum of half a litre of water for few minutes. Turn cooking board off and add spinach leaves. Let is stim under pot's hat for a moment and then mix smooth with blender. After desired consistance is achieved add in white cooking sauce, salt and pepper. You can serve immediately.

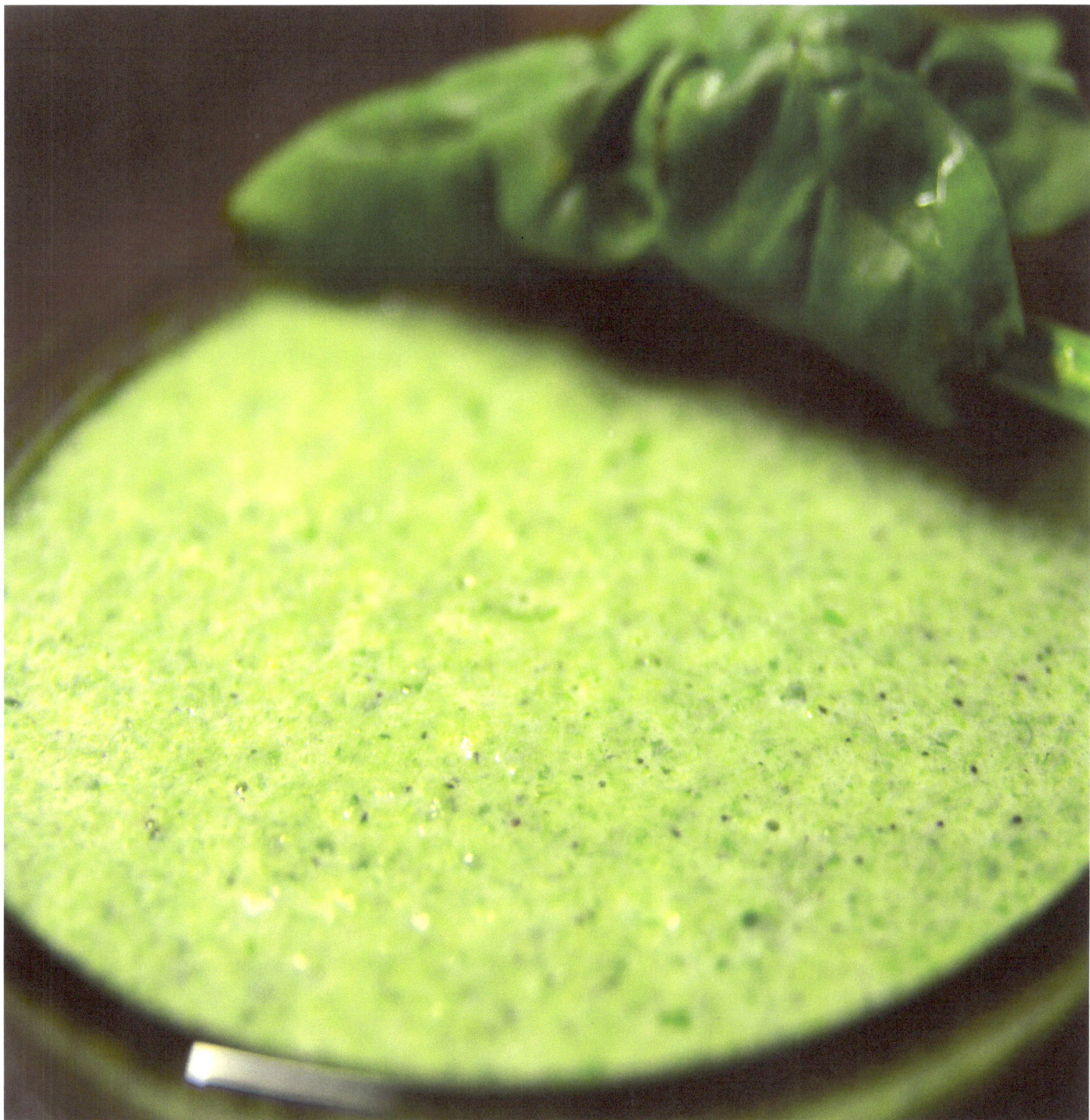

Tom Yum Kung

Tom Yum Kung is the most famous of all Thai soup recipes. Kung stands for prawns in Thai. However it can be as well prepared with chicken (Gai). Should you want an authentic Thai soup this is the one! Featuring all four of the famous Thai spices - salty, sour, sweet and spicy - this Tom Yum Kung recipe provides a pungent and happening feast of flavors with every bite. An excellent remedy for a cold or flu bug, this spicy Thai soup will instantly clear your sinuses and warm you up if you dare to add a bit more chilli. It's also highly nutritious and is sure to impress at any dinner party.

Ingredients:

- 1 galangal (Thai style of ginger - harder to process)
- 5 pieces of fresh chilli padi
- 3 stalks of lemon grass
- tom yam paste (sorry this formlula doesn't cover preparation of this paste)
- 300g of king size prawns (can be of regular size but bigger the better)
- 2 onions
- generous handful of fresh shiitake mushrooms
- fresh coriander
- 3 tomatoes

Method:

First cut all ingredients as follows to ease and speed up cooking. Galangal, lemon grass, and chilli padi will come in first so make sure you have these pieces on separate plate. De-seed chilli padi. Cut onions to quarters, same goes with tomatoes and shiitake mushrooms. Leave these in one bowl ready to be added in. Chop coriander and prepare on table for everyone to garnish themselves since not everyone likes coriander's exotic taste. Choose a big enough pot and put in a bit of oil with tom yum paste. When it starts reacting to heat add all hard ingredients such as lemon grass, galangal and chilli padi. Let it stir for a while and once you can't stand the sharpness of chilli anymore pour over slightly more than half a litre of water. To speed it up it could be boiled already in kettle. When it starts to boil put in all the other ingredients except prawns and let it boil for few minutes. When it looks yummy enough turn the cooking board off and add in prawns. Let it there to boil prawns as well and serve immediately. Should you want to have it solo as main bite you may consider to prepare rice aside (jasmine rice) to support this extraordinary soup.

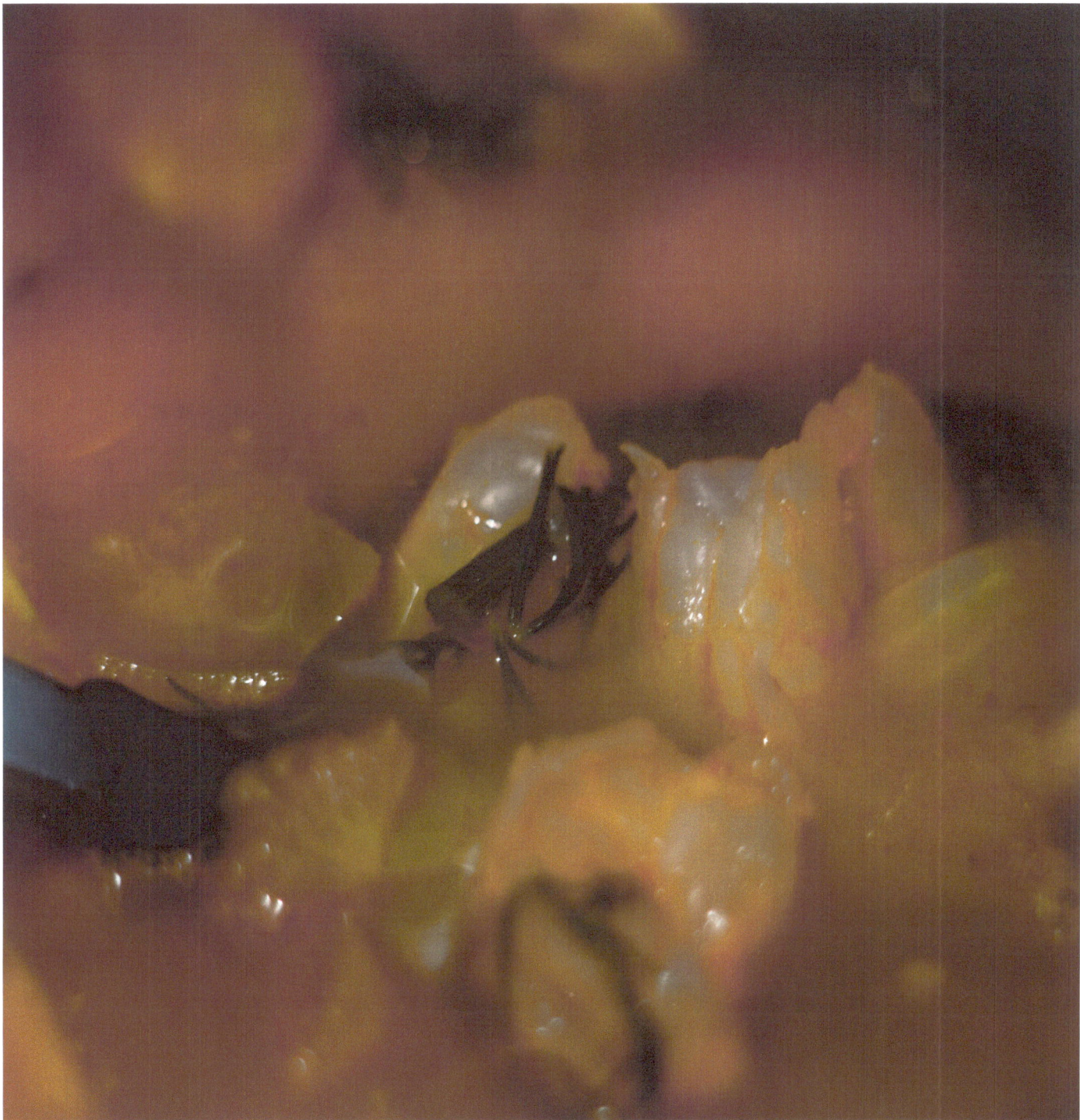

ABC Soup

My wife evidently grew up drinking ABC soup. ABC soup is easy and simple to cook yet taste healthy and delicious! I have no idea why this soup is called ABC. My guess it's because it's simple and easy as ABC and it take no time to cook. It is kid friendly soup too if you hold back pepper.

Ingredients:

- onion
- tomatoes
- chicken meat (having bones is better taste)
- carrot
- potatoes

Method:

Cut all ingredients as follows to speed up cooking. Don't bother with any fine cutting just pieces will do. Leave all in one bowl ready to be added in except tomatoes those will be added last. Start to boil chicken meat, when you see it is oily a bit and boiling you may add all cuts except tomatoes. Let it boil over medium heat for some 10 minutes as if you boil potatoes. Before the end put in tomatoes and turn off the heat. Let it simmer there for few minutes. Add salt and pepper to taste and serve.

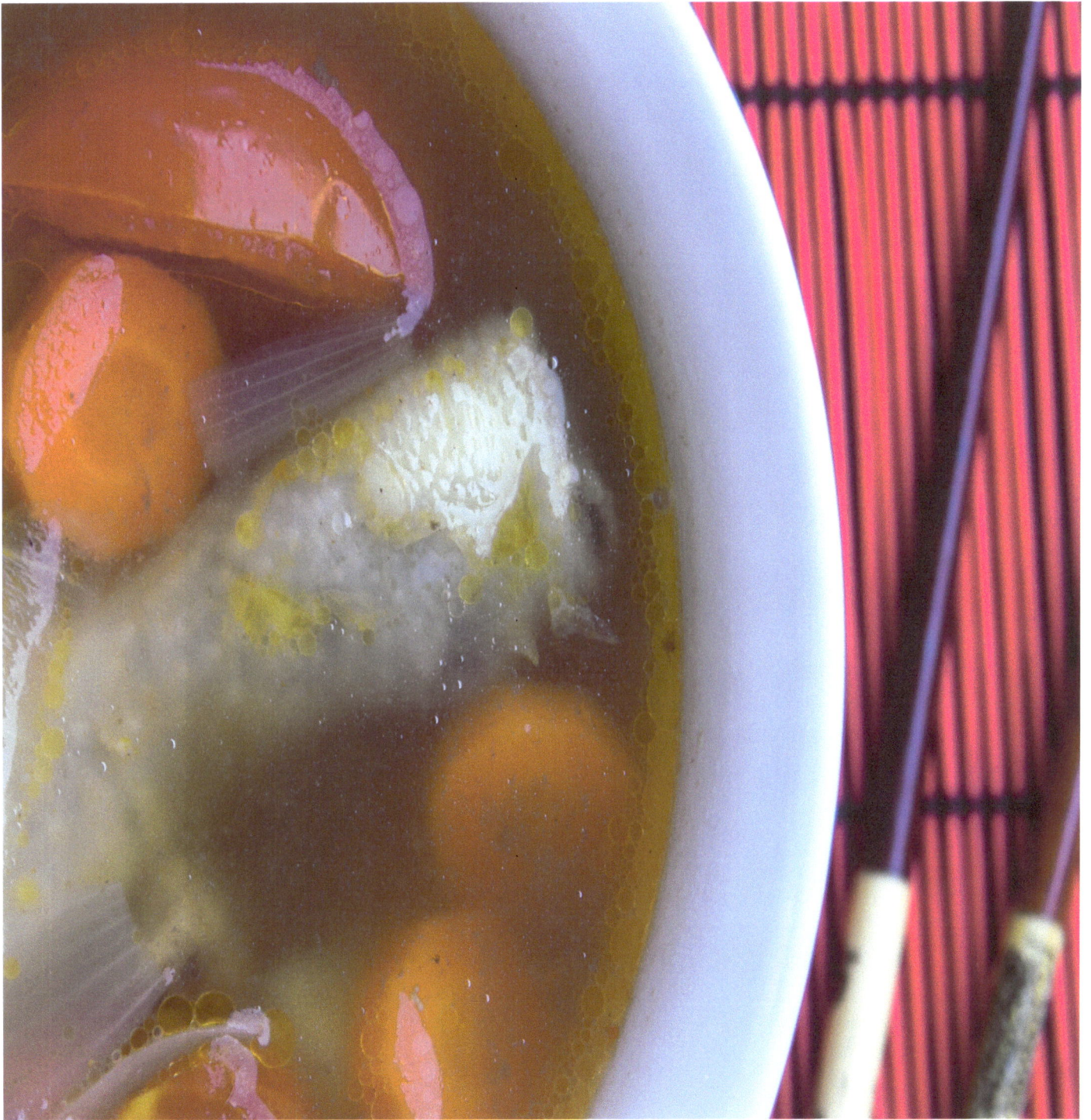

Dill soup

If you're looking for a soup that bridges the seasons, this comforting dish fits the bill. An ample amount of potatoes makes it a satisfying dinner, while the lemon and dill brighten the soup's flavor and give a nod to summer.

Ingredients:

- 3 potatoes
- bunch of fresh dill
- white sauce for cooking
- a piece of butter
- two eggs
- vinegar

Method:

Boil potatoes first but make sure they are not completely done. Finish boiling when they are still hard and transfer them without its water into a new pot. Heat again with fresh water and just before boil point add in white sauce, dill, butter, salt and sugar (yeah right you hear correctly sugar). Turn off cooking board and put in two poached egg. Stir gently so that they keep together. Don't overboil since dill would loose its brisk green colour. Serve with vinegar at everyone's disposal to let them finish for their own taste buds.

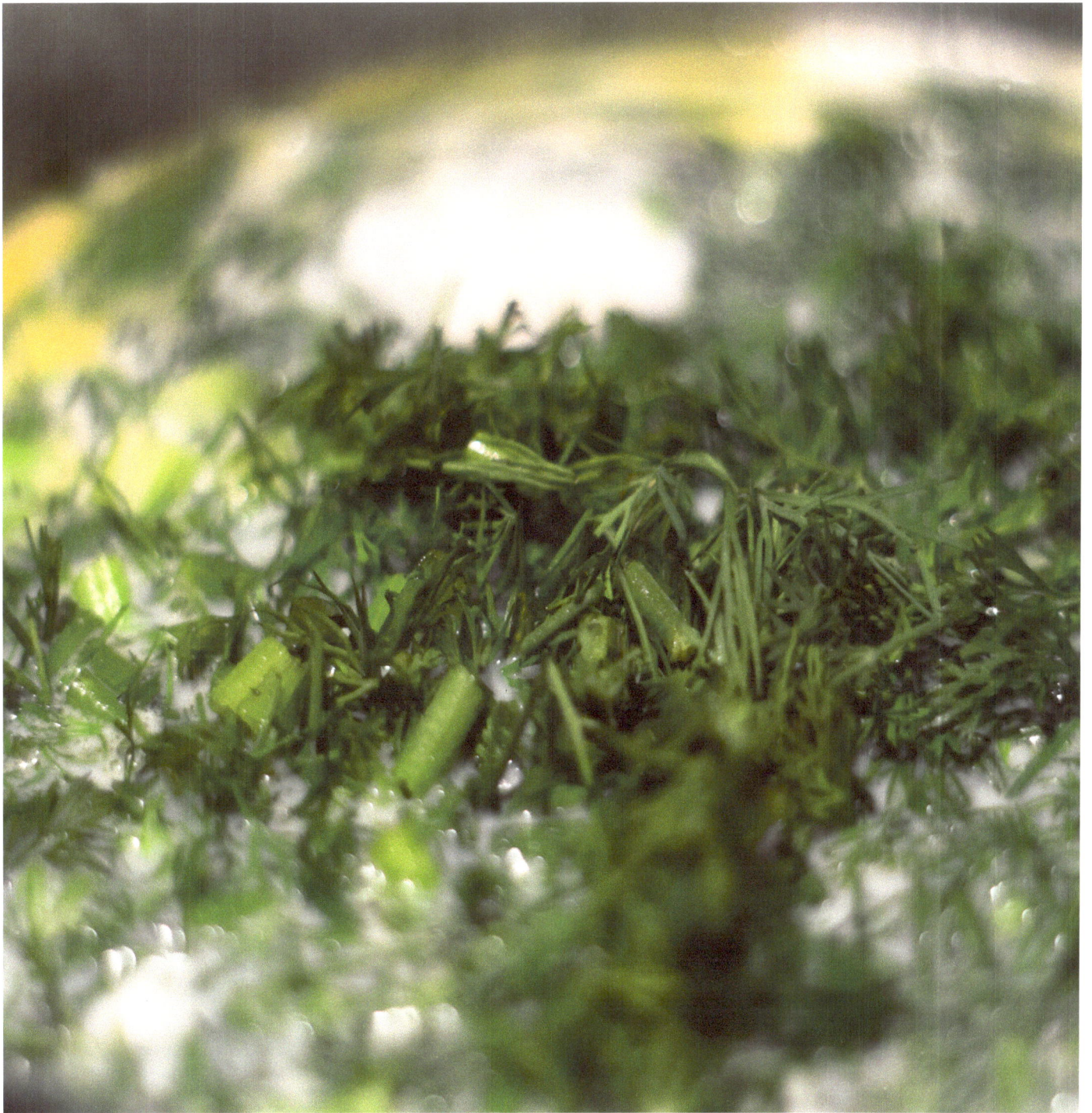

Auxiliary

Here you may find combination of snacks, brunch, desserts, starters or whatever you want to call it. Simply those bites they didn't fit into any category above we gather them here. So are you up to smoothie or garlic paste to keep in fridge for the right occation? Your choice. So enjoy it!

Garlic paste

Garlic is an important ingredient in a great deal of worldwide cuisine, however buying a paste in grocery shop you basically buy a lot of unwanted salt. Here's how to make garlic paste which thanks to olive oil going to last long in fridge.. .read on to add its spicy flavor to your kitchen.

Ingredients:

- at least 2 bulb of garlic. Try to buy local one instead of tasteless 'chinese' garlic.
- olive oil

Method:

Take out the cloves of garlic and peel off the skin.Put them in a blender and add just a little of oil (eventually try to cover those cloves in their half, but put less first you can add later on). Blend into a smooth paste. Transfer this paste into an air tight container and store in the refrigerator. Usually this paste can be stored in the refrigerator for up to 3 weeks.

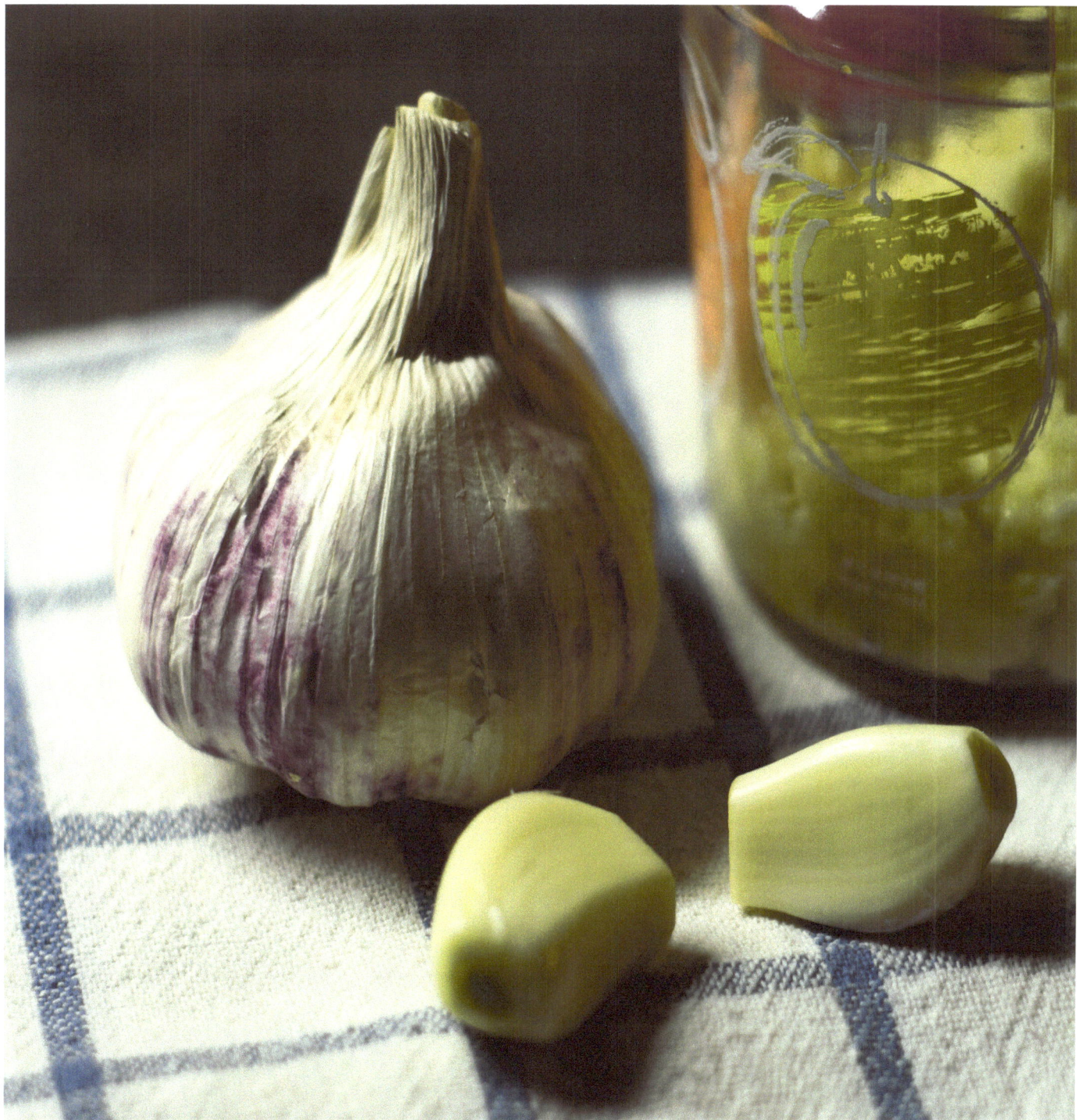

Strawberry Smoothie

Strawberry smoothies are delicious, healthy, and last but not least easy to make. They can also be a fantastic party treat or a refreshing afternoon snack.

Ingredients:

- 12 pieces of strawberries
- two plain yogurt

Method:

Pour strawberries into the blender, optionally add ice and yogurt. Plain yogurt will impart a tarter flavor and will allow the fresh fruit to come through more. Blend for about 5 seconds, pause, then blend again. Repeat until mixed.

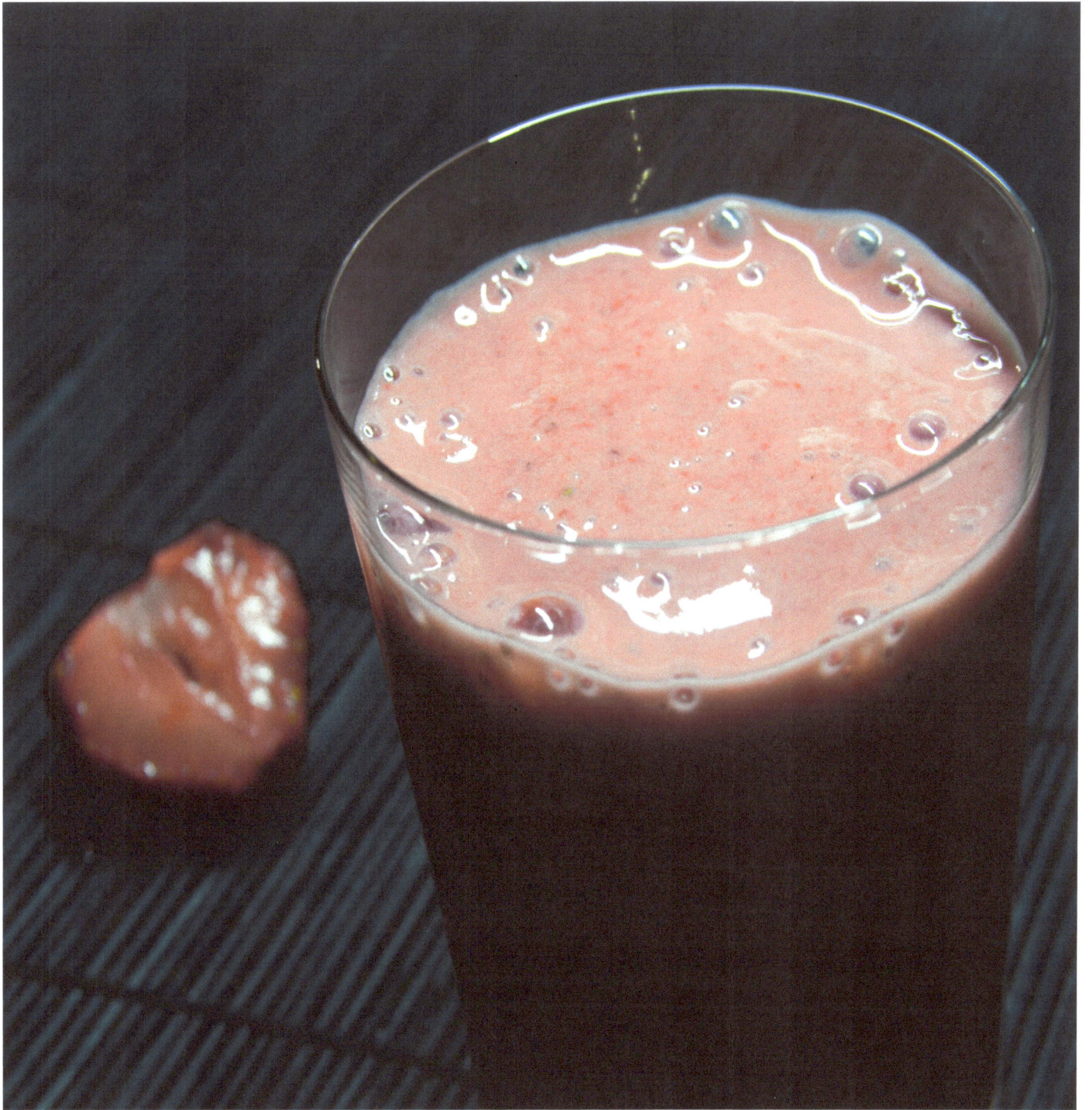

Lemongrass drink

Looking for a change from sugary fruit juice? Try this nicely balanced fragrant lemongrass drink. Add some ice cubes and it's perfect for cooling down on a hot summer's day. Serve it hot and it makes good company in chilly weather. Lemon is optional as it is stronger taste than lemongrass.

Ingredients:

- 2 stalks of fresh lemongrass
- 1.5 litre of water
- optionally half of lemon

Method:

Boil water and while boiling crush the lemon grass with something heavy or use knife to squeze the stalk. Wash properly and peel off any leaves that have turned brown just for hygiene purposes. Peel and cut the lemon, put all into pot and pour over with boiled water. Serve once flavour enlarges and water is not hot anymore. During summer's days just don't boil water and use ice cubes instead.

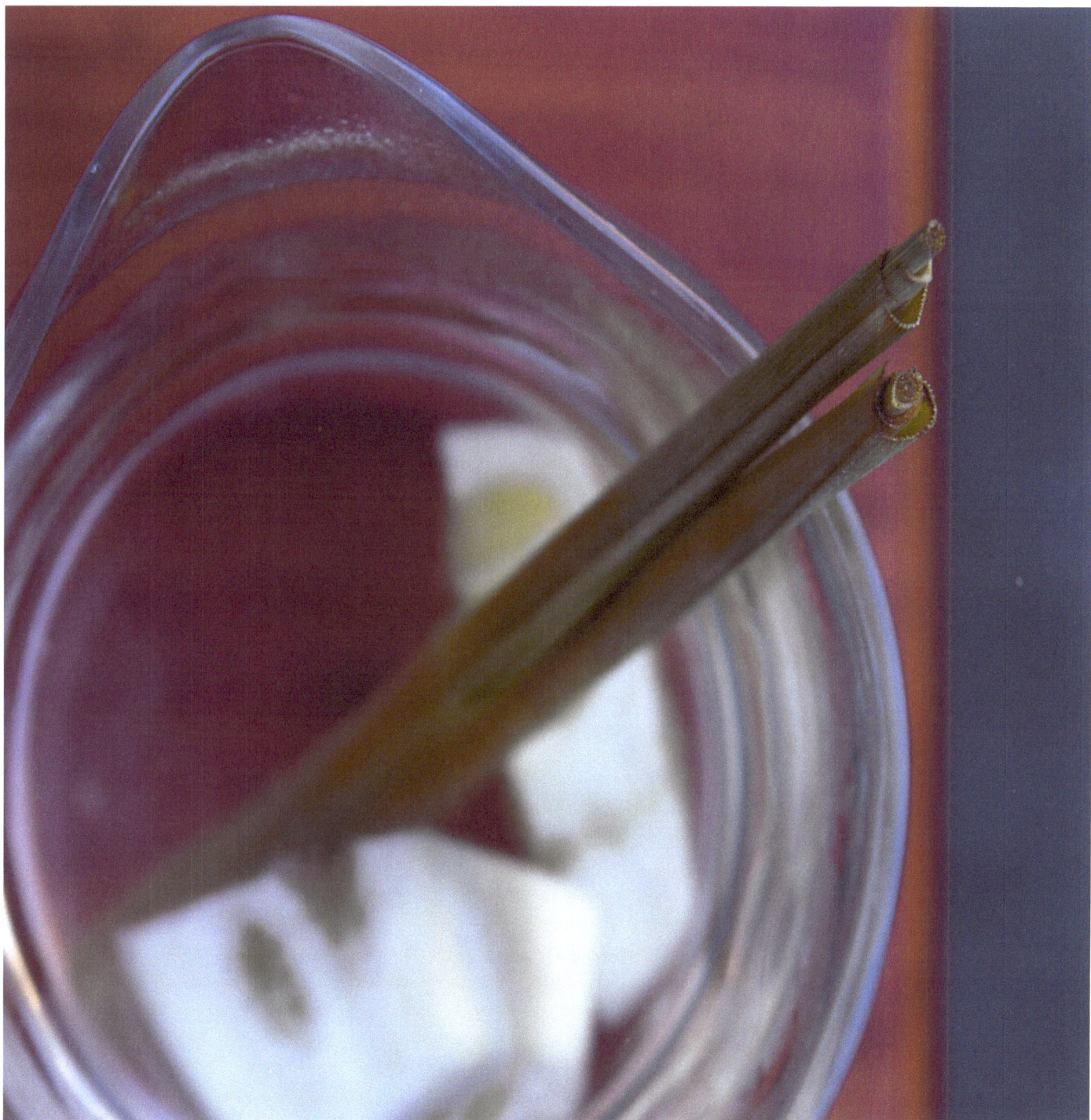

Guacamole

Guacamole, a dip made from avocados, is originally from Mexico. All you really need for guacamole is ripe avocados and salt. After that, a little lime - a splash of acidity to balance the richness of the avocado. Then comes chopped green vege like coriander, chiles, onion, and garlic, if you want.

The trick to a perfect guacamole is using good, ripe avocados. Check for ripeness by gently pressing the outside of the avocado. If there is no give, the avocado is not ripe yet and will not taste good. If there is a little give, the avocado is ripe. If there is a lot of give, the avocado may be past ripe and not good. In this case, taste test first before using.

Ingredients:

- 2 ripe avocados
- juice of one lime
- 1 tablespoon of oil
- 1 onion
- 1 garlic clove

Method:

Cut the avocadoes in half lenghtways and twist the 2 halfes in opposite directions to separate then lift out the seed. Peel, then roughly chop the avocado and place it into a non-metallic bowl. Squeeze over the lime juice and add oil. Mash the avocadoes with fork until desired consistency is achieved - either chunky or smooth. Blend in the fine chopped onion, chilli, garlic, coriander and season to taste with salt and pepper.
Serve immediately to avoid discoloration with tortilla chips and garnished with fresh dill springs

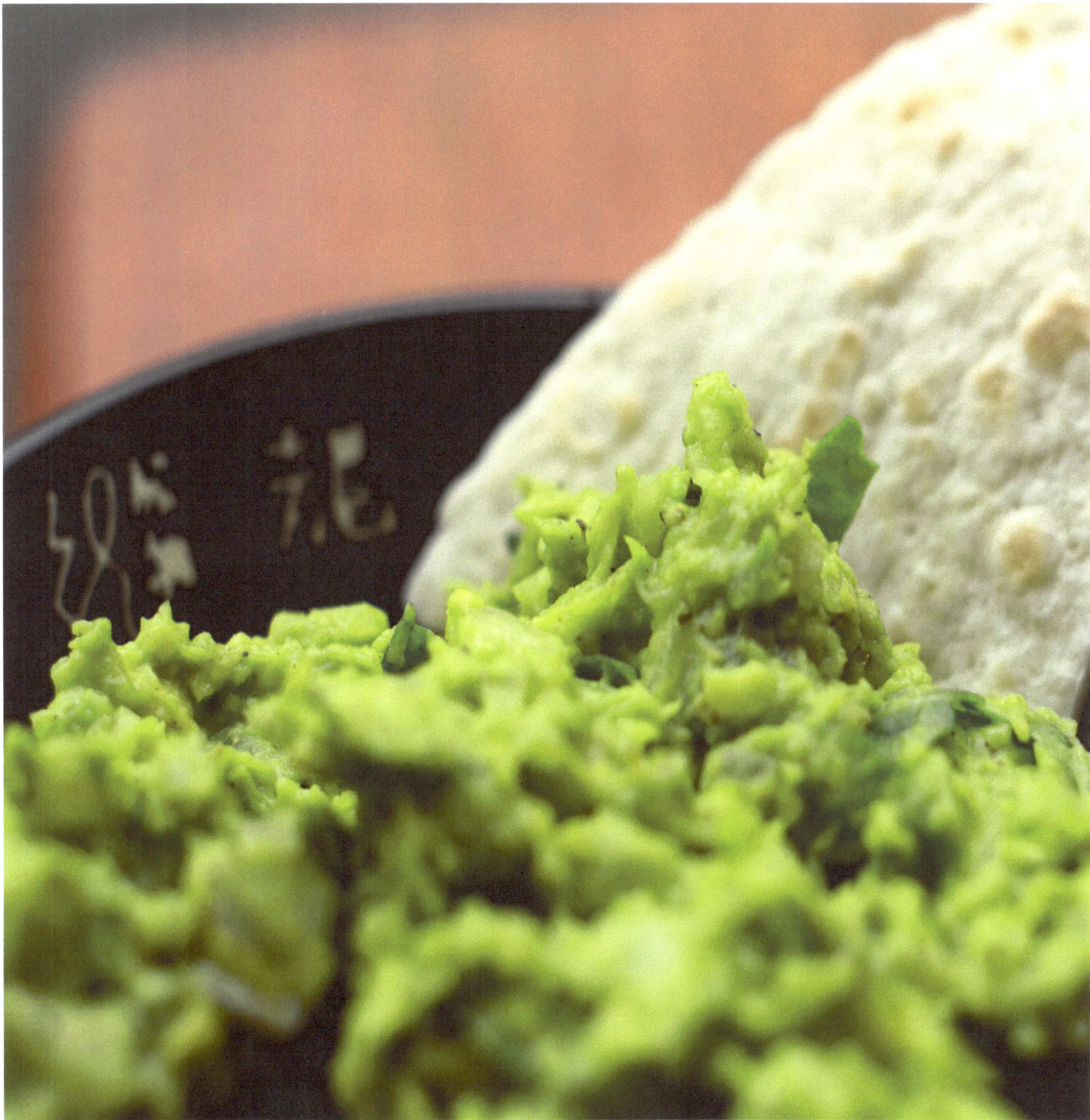

Breakfast eggs variations

We came across eggs few times already, so we don't need to explain why do we choose egg as one of basic part of our approach however here let's try to be a bit more creative with presentation this time.

Ingredients:

- 4 eggs
- 2 whole wheat bun
- few slices of a big sweet pepper

Method:

Cut two slices from the thick part of sweet pepper and put then on pan, then do fried egg within the border of pepper. Transfer on top of the bun when done. A poached egg is an egg that has been cooked by poaching, that is, in simmering liquid. This method of preparation is favored because of a very consistent and predictable result can be attained with precise timing, as the boiling point of water removes the temperature variable from the cooking process. Boil water and once boiling decrease the heat and gently open en egg into the water so that it will keep as much together. Let it boil for a minute or two and transfer to bun. This is correctly prepared only when bitten egg yolk is still watery. Season with pepper and salt and enjoy.

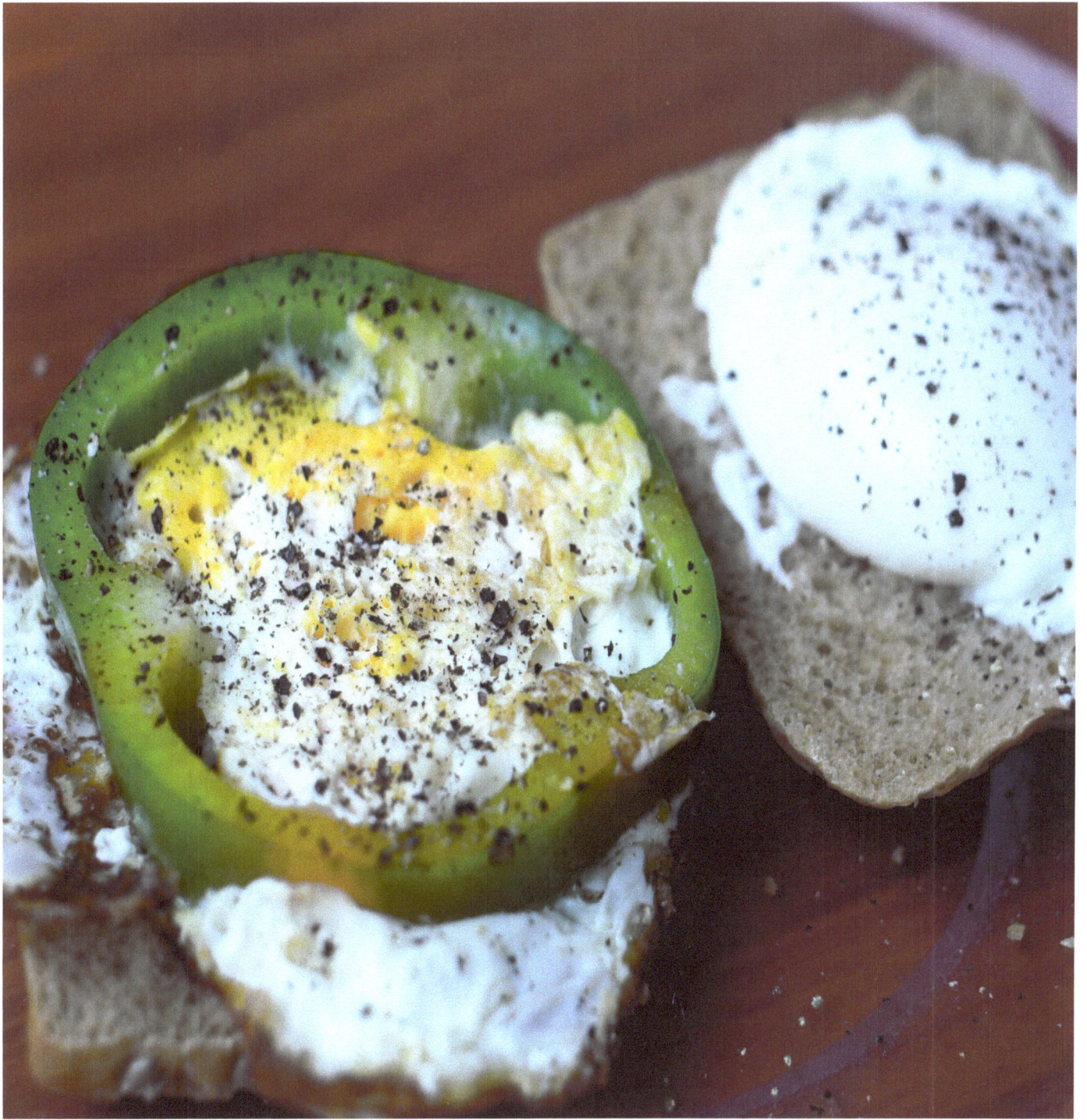

Jacked potato

Over internet there will be plenty of variations how to do a perfect jacked potato so we just have one here since he like it the most. As with sausages, the world is divided between those who prick their jacket potatoes, and those who don't. We don't, we rather use inner part of potato for mixture. This dish is easy but will hardly take you less than 30 minutes. So please be patient it is worth waiting.

Ingredients:

- 2 fatty potatoes
- 1 tbsp chopped fresh parsley or chives
- bacon
- spread cheese
- garlic

Method:

Pre-boil potatoes until the point they are still not done but not that hard anymore. Meanwhile prepare the mixture. Chop fresh parsley or chives mix them with finely cut garlic and spread cheese. Mix properly and wait for potatoes to be done. When potatoes are ready put them aside of heat and cool them down with cold water. Use spoon to dig inner part of potatoes and mix is with already done mixture. Stuff potatoes and put them to oven for approximately 200 degrees for duration of 30 min. After that put a piece of bacon to each top part and put it back to oven. As soon as you like the colour of bacon you can serve.

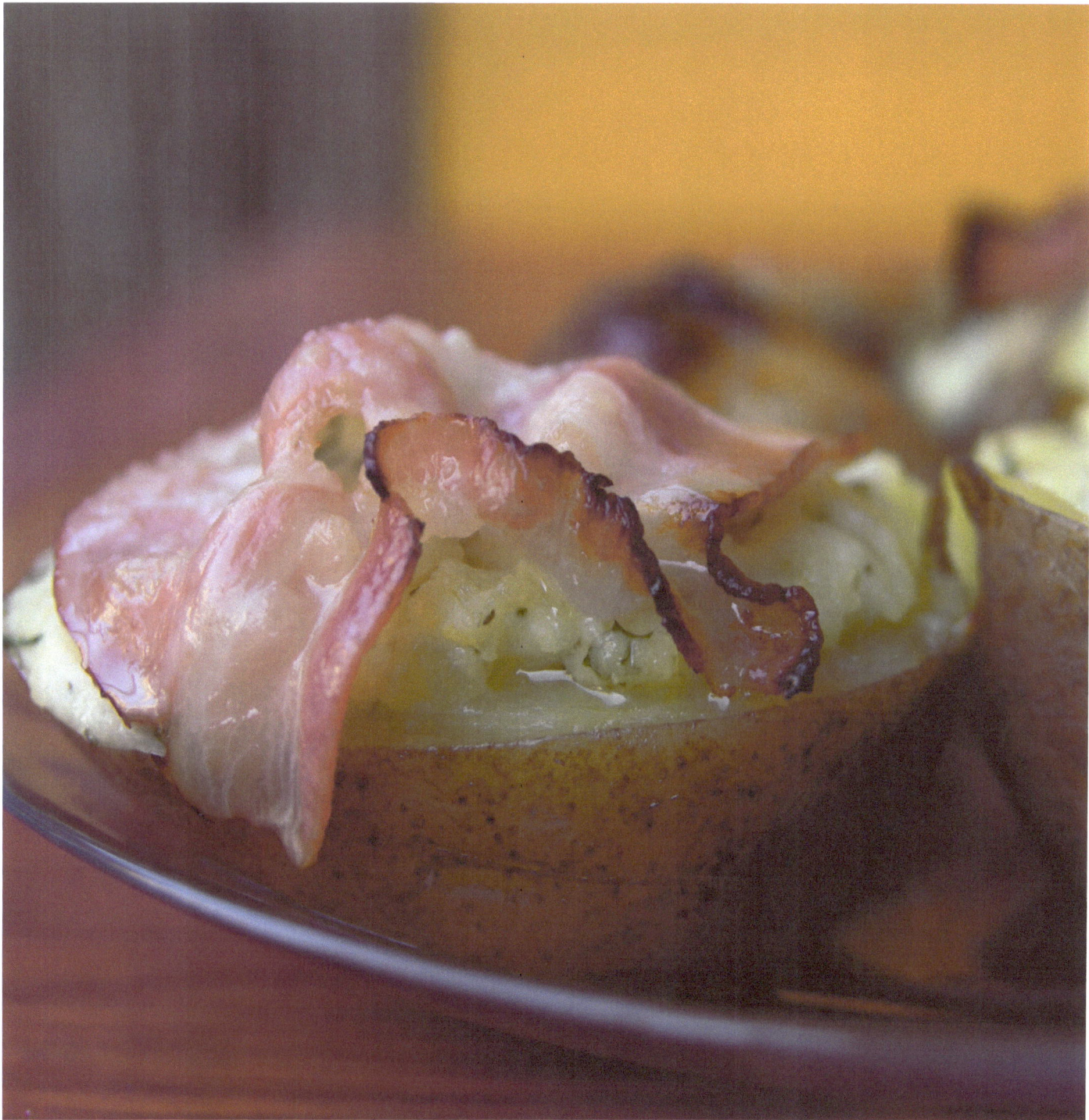

Sweet pepper and cheese grill

Sweet peppers don't come in just red and green anymore, nor are they just different colors of bell peppers. Yellow, orange, and purple peppers are fairly commonplace, not to mention the range of sizes and varieties within the red pepper world beyond sweet bells. Almost no matter what colour they are grassy in flavor and super-crunchy in texture. Putting them into oven with a bit of cheese makes surprisingly nice light dinner.

Ingredients:

- 3 sweet pepper
- 100 g of edam cheese

Method:

Cut sweet pepper into some reasonable size pieces for you to be able to put cheese on it later. Peel out inner part that is full of seeds, and then put them all onto stove pan. Place a slice of cheese on top of each piece and let it grill in oven for some ~15 minutes depends on how crunchy you want to have them. Eventually towards the end of grilling swith program to grill so that you will gain slightly burned out surface. Enjoy just like that or with a glass of white wine.

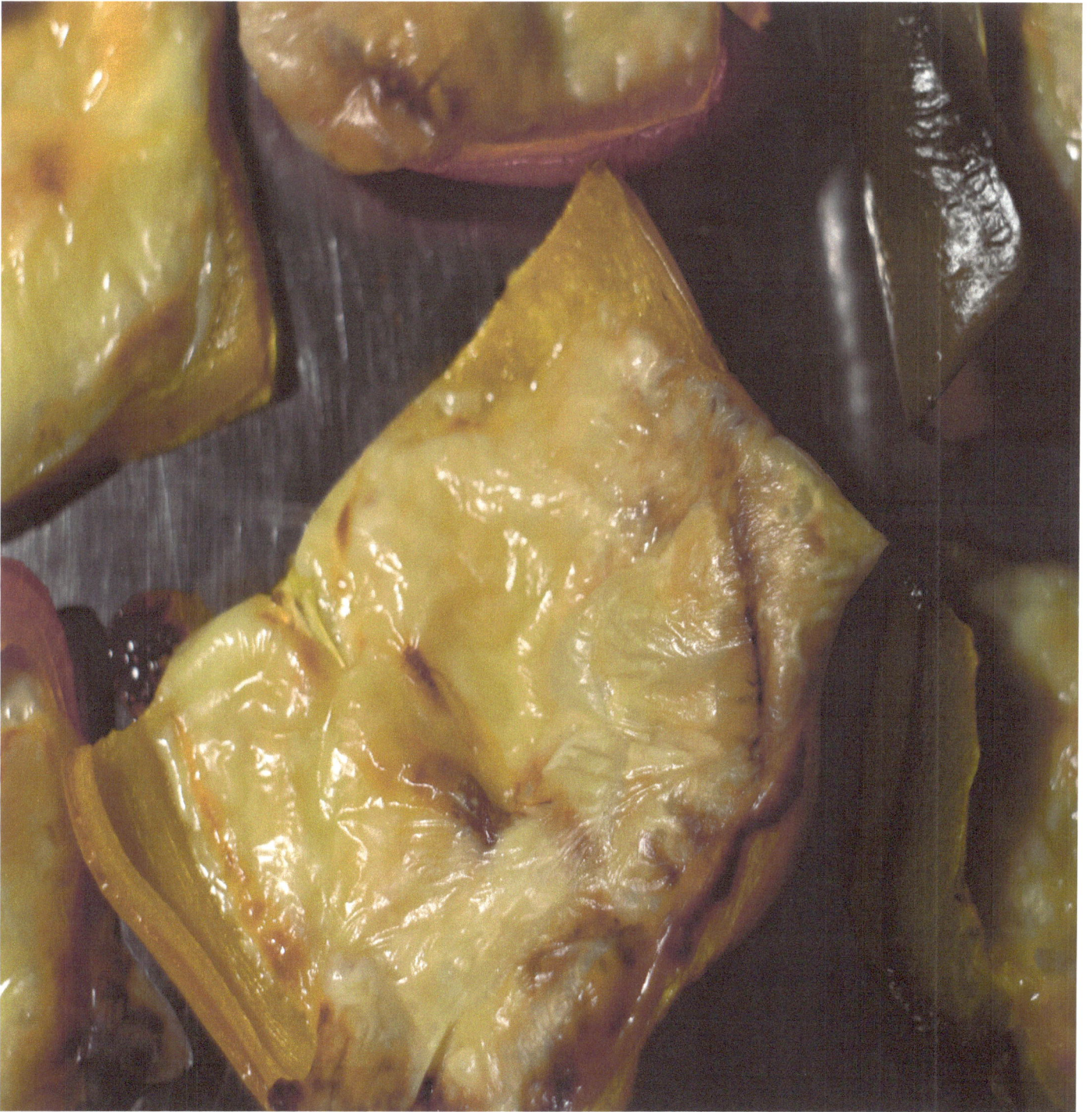

Mint tea

Fresh mint tea is one of the ways I know that spring is here for sure. Because out of all herbs out there in our small garden, the mint is always the first one to leaf out, and just like that, winter is gone and summer is just around the corner. And one the best way to celebrate (especially on those spring days when there is still a little chill in the air) is a warm, sweet-smelling cup of the easiest tea in the world to make. Most tea will fight stress, and mint is no exception. Mint tea is typically used to alleviate digestive trouble. It can calm an upset stomach, relieve nausea and diminish gas. Drinking mint tea will also help remove dangerous bacteria from the digestive system and prevent cold and flu. Along with easing digestive trouble, mint tea provides a number of diverse health benefits. Mint can freshen breath and is useful against colds because of its ability to decongest stuffy sinuses and reduce chest pain. Mint can aid in maintaining a healthy weight, since mint leaves help break down fat cells in the body.

Ingredients:

- few stalks with mint leaves
- water

Method:

Usually, I would grap few stalks with leaves for one kettle of water which has 1.7 l . After the leaves are properly washed, you can either crush them in mortar or at least tear them into half (don't use metal kitchenware though) and pour over boiling water. Wait for few minutes once all that mind fragrance and colour makes up your tea and then just relax having one cup in your hand.

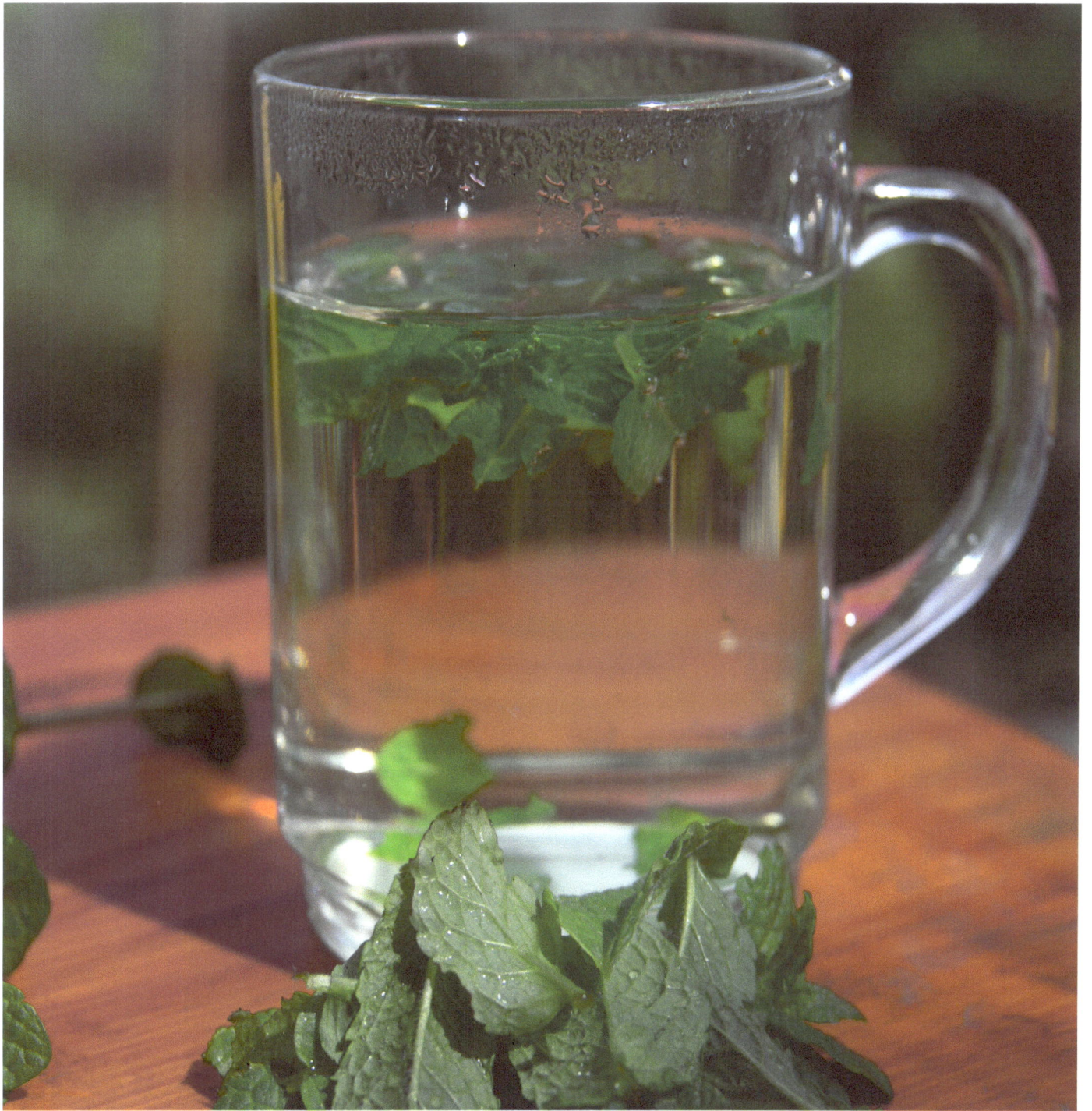

www.ingramcontent.com/pod-product-compliance
Lightning Source LLC
Chambersburg PA
CBHW060813270326
41929CB00002B/25